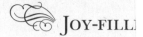 Joy-Fill

In *JOY-spirations for Caregivers,* Annetta and Karen wisely come alongside fellow caregivers with sensitivity, compassion, humor, practical advice, and most important, the strengthening word of "The Ultimate Caregiver," God.

—**Janet Thompson,** CA
Speaker and author of *Dear God, They Say It's Cancer:
A Companion Guide for Women on the Breast Cancer Journey*

For those struggling with the "Why's?" of caregiving, this book brings comfort, insight, and encouragement from God and from the authors' own understanding and solid advice based on their personal experiences.

—**Marlys Taege,** WI
Retired Corporate Affairs Administrator
Bethesda Lutheran Homes and Services

JOY-spirations for Caregivers offers nourishment to the caregiver in God's Word, provides humor in the moments of anxiety, and gives hope for tomorrow.

—**Terry Lee Kieschnick,** MO
Motivational Speaker

Annetta and Karen reveal the questions and frustrations of caregivers, but they also provide helpful guides along this very challenging and rewarding journey. They are right on target!

—**Bob Willis,** OK
Southern Baptist Minister, Bereavement Coordinator
Hospice of Oklahoma County

Caregivers will feel less alone, more understood, and greatly encouraged by this creative, honest look at the challenges and rewards of caregiving.

—**Steve Siler,** TN
Director, Music for the Soul

JOY-spirations for Caregivers is a wonderful resource for caregivers and for those who love and support them. The book is interwoven with scripture, poems, JOYtoons, and meditations from the heart and experience of caregivers.

—**Jan Wendorf**, WI
President, Lutheran Women in Mission

Caregivers often feel alone and inadequate to do the tasks required of them. Their many concerns are addressed in a practical and biblical manner. These short reads are perfect for the busy caregiver.

—**Shirley Braddock**, FL
Retired Oncology Nurse

Reading *JOY-spirations for Caregivers* reminded me of conversations I had with God while caring for my mother. I wish I could have read this book then.

—**Marcia Schnorr**, IL
Coordinator, LCMS Parish Nursing

As a caregiver, these insights, faith-boosters, and joyful thoughts relieve my stress and point me to God.

—**Kathy Collard Miller**, CA
Speaker and author, *Women of the Bible:
the Smart Guide to the Bible*

JOY-spirations for Caregivers reaches out with eternal, life-saving words of comfort. This is the perfect gift for a caregiver.

—**Mary Hilgendorf**, Ph.D., WI
Ambassador for Women's Leadership Institute
Concordia University Wisconsin

The writers know what it means to feel the loneliness and guilt that often accompanies caregiving. This book will give them the assurance of God's unending love and presence in their lives.

—**Rev. Gerald Matzke**, OH
LCMS Pastor and former OH District Human Care Chm.

JOY-spirations for Caregivers is a well-written and delightful book and a must read for any caregiver.

—**Jackie Holland**, TX
TV Host, Author, Speaker, and Caregiver

Annetta and Karen will reach through the pages, give you a hug, and provide encouragement in your caregiving journey.

—**Sherri Goss**, CFP, GA
Financial Advisor and Author of *My Life Book*

JOY-spirations for Caregivers offers parents nurturing their children with special needs a dose of inspiration and insight when they need it most . . . they're not alone.

—**Janet Mitchell**, CA
Caregiver, Speaker and Author of
It Just Takes One . . . to make a difference in your world

Pick up this book . . . pause, breathe deeply, and take in the fresh air of renewal.

—**Phyllis Wallace**, MO
Host of "Woman to Woman" Talk Radio

JOY-spirations
for
Caregivers

JOY-spirations
for
Caregivers

Dialogues with God of Hope and Encouragement

Annetta Dellinger
&
Karen Boerger

Illustrated by George L. Richardson

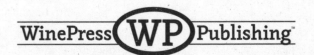

WinePress **WP** Publishing

WinePress Publishing (PO Box 428, Enumclaw, WA 98022) functions only as book publisher. As such, the ultimate design, content, editorial accuracy, and views expressed or implied in this work are those of the author.

Illustrated by George L. Richardson: www.artofencouragement.org.

ISBN 13: 978-1-60615-026-9
ISBN 10: 1-60615-026-X
Library of Congress Catalog Card Number: 2009936184

Thank You, Lord, for giving us Your strength
during our caregiving seasons.
We dedicate this book to our special loved ones:
Annetta Dellinger—Luther and Lena Heigle
Karen Boerger—Warren and Helen Gorden, Joann Gorden,
Tilda Boerger, and Florence Teegarden

Our JOY-filled Thanks!

We want to thank all our family and friends for blessing us with their encouragement, prayers, and support. We especially thank our husbands—John Dellinger and Marvin Boerger—for their patience and encouragement. We love you!

A JOYful thank-you to our readers, editors, encouragers, and prayer partners:

Dawn Boerger, Arleen and Rev. Gordon Bohlmann, Shirley Braddock, Cathy Burns, Sue Ann and Mark Dillahunt, Sherri Goss, Jacquie Ingles, Carmen Leal, Ida Luebke, Rev. Gerald Matzke, Tom and Amy McCarthy, Janet Lynn Mitchell, Rachel and Rita Rinehart, Sharon Richardson, Rev. Robert Willis, and our praying friends.

We are grateful to John Dellinger for his excellent technical support.

Praise God from whom all blessings flow!

Annetta and Karen

Contents

A Word of Welcome to You, Our Dear Caregiver!

Why are the words *"real* JOY" laced throughout a book for caregivers? Isn't the life of a caregiver exhausting, stressful, and lonely? What about the constant challenges and changes? *JOY in a book for caregivers? Yes!*

Real JOY is permanent when rooted in God and is quite different from the temporary happiness of the world. God's presence is the caregiver's only sustaining and unchanging source of strength. His faithfulness gives us confidence to cope with the day-to-day challenges. *God is our caregiver!*

We, the authors, have experienced a total of eight caregiving seasons. The JOY of God's presence was the calm in chaos through our tears and fears. We are now vastly enriched from this journey. We grew stronger in our prayer lives and deeper in our relationships with the Lord. We also learned how it is easy to love someone when things are going well, but that the true test of love is being able to show it when you are exhausted from the never-ending struggles of caring for a loved one.

You are God's hands to your loved one, dear caregiver. He wants to talk with you and does through the thirty-six topics in *JOY-spirations for Caregivers*. He will embrace you with

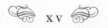

assurance and hope as you sit at His feet and are encouraged by His words that address your many gut-wrenching concerns. You will connect with people from the Bible whose life situations are similar to yours, and you will see God's faithfulness through all generations!

In addition, the meditations in *JOY-spirations for Caregivers* will strengthen you with God's promises. You will read stories woven with practical life applications and with guidance for the various situations you may face.

We know, dear caregiver, that you have little time for yourself. That's why *JOY-spirations for Caregivers* contains short, power-packed, and uplifting sections based on Scripture. You can read the book cover to cover or enjoy individual pages at random.

As you have the opportunity, please share the book with others. It will give them a new perspective on caregiving. Encourage everyone to enjoy the light-hearted but insightful JOYtoons. Remember, there is healing in humor.

Silent hero, our greatest desire is that this book will be an encouragement for you to know that you are never alone and that the *real* JOY of God's presence will be your strength in this journey!

Annetta and Karen

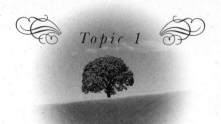

Realities of
Caregiving

Dear God,

This is not what I signed up to do! I never pictured my life
   this way.
   Are you *really* sure, God, that You planned for *me* to be
      a *caregiver?*

In my heart I know that Your plans are always good, so
   forgive me for questioning You.
   Right now, the reality of being a caregiver is that it's
      never-ending.
   I'm *overwhelmed!*

I feel *unprepared* to deal with the constant changes in my
   loved one's health, and
   I have very little time for myself. You know me, Lord;
      I love to plan ahead.
   I have control over *nothing* now!

I am on a constant *guilt* trip.
   When I'm with my loved one, I feel guilty because
      I can't meet my other responsibilities.

Then, when I am doing other things, I feel guilty
because I'm not with my loved one.

I'm stressed, exhausted, and afraid.
I'm beginning to resent the people I love.
I'm lonely for what my life used to be, and
I miss my friends.
I'm angry at myself for not being more gracious and
patient.

I'm so glad I can be honest with You about my emotions.
I don't think anyone else would understand.

Lord, I need You!

I'm listening . . .

I love You,
Your Caregiving Child

Praise be to the God and Father of our Lord Jesus Christ,
the Father of compassion and the God of all comfort,
who comforts us in all our troubles, so that you can
comfort those in any trouble with the comfort
we ourselves have received from God.
—2 Corinthians 1:3–4

Realities of Caregiving

My Child,

Come. Come into My arms as I comfort and embrace you
with My unfailing love.
> Because *I* am always with you, you'll be strengthened
> to meet every need in your caregiving *season.*

Caregiving, like the seasons in nature, may not be brief,
but it is for a limited time.
> Remember how you watched the flower bulbs grow
> and bloom after the hard
> winter?

> Seasons in nature and in your
> life may continually change,
> but I will *never* abandon you.

**My child, I am
your caregiver!**

> My grace will *always* be suf-
> ficient. My child,
> *I am your caregiver*!

I know how heavy your heart is from
the realities you face. Please believe that . . .
> I know how your blood pressure soared when you
> heard the test results.
> I know how brokenhearted you are from watching
> your loved one struggle.
> I stood by your side as you leaned against the wall
> crying and thinking about giving up.

I am a merciful Father and the source of all comfort.
> My child, I will *comfort you* so that you can *comfort others.*

You'll find hope and assurance of My faithfulness as you
read about Joseph in your Bible.
> He wondered if anything good would come out of . . .
> > ✍ the time his brothers threw him in the pit and
> > then sold him.
> > ✍ his life in prison.
> > ✍ his palace lifestyle.

Joseph knew about realities and found *hope* in My
  presence.
I didn't betray Joseph, even though he may not have
  understood how I was caring for him.
    I didn't promise to spare anyone from day-to-day
      challenges, but you can *trust Me* to stand beside you,
      teach you, and strengthen you!
    Use this caregiving season as another opportunity to
      grow closer to Me.

Joseph learned the secret of true JOY, which goes much
  deeper than temporary happiness,
    because spiritual JOY comes through *our relationship.*
      That's an eternal promise!
    My Son, Jesus Christ, proved My everlasting love for
      you when He died on the cross and rose again.
    That's why you can walk boldly through the realities in
      your caregiving season!

My child, I am *your* caregiver.

I love you!
God

May the God of hope fill you with all joy and peace as you
trust in him, so that you may overflow with hope
by the power of the Holy Spirit.
—Romans 15:13

Today, walk in the JOY of God's Word!

Read Joseph's story in Genesis 37–45.

Many are the plans in a man's heart,
but it is the LORD's purpose that prevails.
—Proverbs 19:21

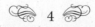

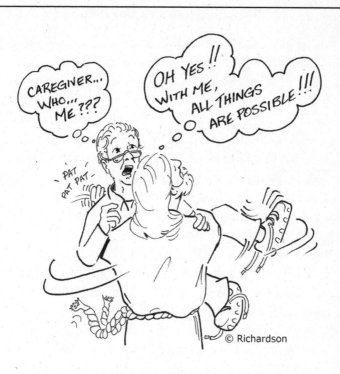

Team One

It cannot be,
    this is not me,
        Oh, Lord, this can't be fun.

The joy to care,
    will be your share,
        when we team up as one.
                    —*George Richardson*

Biblical Inspiration: Mark 10:27

❧ Emotions in a Box ❧

An imaginary, old, wooden box sat on the top shelf in my closet just waiting to be opened at the appropriate time. The gift tag read: "Caregiver." I (Karen) wondered whom it was for. I didn't know anyone with that name.

My first caregiving role was when my husband was diagnosed with depression. During his lengthy illness, the lid of that wooden box suddenly flew open and emotions and moods erupted, seeping into everything I did. Yes, I was a caregiver, and I didn't like what that box had to share with me. After all, I am a Christian. We are supposed to be kind, patient, and caring, aren't we? But I wasn't!

Anger and *frustration* raised their ugly heads when my husband took no interest in our family. He would just sit in a chair with a blank, sad face and often would spend much of the day in a deep sleep in his chair while shutting out the world. The burden on the children to care for the large hog and dairy farm was *overwhelming*. I was worried about them, and to survive, I built a wall around my heart to protect myself from being hurt.

Often I would feel *guilt* creep in when I lashed out with harsh words or when I had to use tough love. Couldn't he do anything for himself? Only God kept me safe as I drove to work through my tears.

Underlying all of this was *fear*. I wondered: *Is this the way it will always be? Will he recover and be the man I married again? Will he take his own life?*

The next caregiving situation was my mother's Alzheimer's disease. This was followed by my stepmother's lung cancer, which came with an unscrupulous caregiver (from the agency that worked with my stepmother's care) who slyly gained favor with my dad and worked to see how much money she could get. Then there was my aunt, who was a long-distance caregiving situation, and my mother-in-law, who was a brief living-at-home one. Oh, the stories I could tell about my experiences! And, yes, the lid flies off that box every time another caregiving experience comes up in my life. I've tried to understand why that is. After all, I learned from my first caregiving experience as well as from the next ones that came along. So why do these emotions from the box bombard me each time?

How grateful I am today that God has led me to see that the old, wooden box that plagued me has been changed to an old, rugged cross—an emblem of suffering and pain. But my pain is nothing in comparison to the pain of my Savior when He took the sins of the world upon Himself and, out of love for all of us, made a way for us to be clean and spotless in the eyes of our Creator.

I praise God that my husband is in good health today. Because I have been able to see a part of the plan that God has designed for me, I am able to encourage others in their caregiving roles. Today, making a difference in other people's lives is my passion because I have experienced what they are going through. In the dark valleys of emotional pain, God has made me stronger and more compassionate. He put me in the potter's kiln and fired me up for His kingdom. This produced a stronger faith in me than I ever had before.

I've learned how important it is to take hold of God's hand and never let go! Daily, He gives me comfort and strength to meet the challenges because He *lives*. He is my everlasting hope. That's your hope, too. That's real JOY!

> *Dear Caregiver,* A technique that helps us to give our emotions to God and leave them there is taken from 2 Kings 4:8–36. It's called "The Keeping Envelope."[1] Write the emotions that

you need help with on pieces of paper and put them in "The Keeping Envelope." Seal it, and ask God to free you from this burden. By relinquishing control, you are yielding to God's grace. You may find, like we did, that in the crisis of faith this leads to a deeper intimacy with God through prayer.

Annetta and Karen

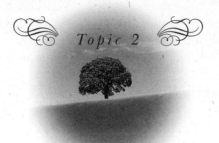

Asking "Why Me?"

Dear God,

Why? Why? Why?

For many years we've been keeping a list of our
    "Retirement Dreams."
        No alarm clocks . . . Hawaii . . . The Swiss Alps . . .
        Always being available when friends or grandchildren
            say, "Come."
        But now, his illness has changed everything.

Why, God? Why?

Where do I begin?
    I've never had to take care of the bills before.
    What if I hit the wrong button on the computer and
        delete our entire account?
    I used to depend on him. Now he depends on me.
    Why did I take all these things for granted?

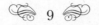

My intentions were good when I planned to make a
notebook to keep important information in,
such as whom to call to fix the furnace or how to
record a program on the TV.
Why did I put that off?

I am ashamed to admit it, but I am really angry with You,
God.
I have to say I resent the loss of our unfilled dreams, and
I'm scared because I don't know if I'll have what it
takes to do this.
How can I do everything?
What would you have me do now?

I am listening . . .

> **I love You,**
> **Your Curious Child**

Show me your ways, O LORD, teach me your paths; guide me
in your truth and teach me, for you are God my Savior,
and my hope is in you all day long.
—Psalm 25:4–5

My Child,

Take a deep breath and relax as you come into My presence.
    Pour out your burdened heart, My child. *I am your
    caregiver,* and I'm waiting for you.

King David didn't tiptoe into My presence but burst into
    My throne room
        and cried out for all the grace and power he needed.
        I encourage you to come boldly, too!

As you spend time with Me, you'll find *endless hope.*
    My Word is a transcript of My love and faithfulness to
    all generations.

In the book of Ruth you'll read about Naomi, who also
    asked, "Why? What should I do now?"
        Naomi's plans changed drastically!
        Soon after her family moved to a new country, her
        husband and two sons died.
        And even though I provided Ruth, a devoted
        daughter-in-law who vowed, "Where you go I will
        go, and where you stay I will stay," Naomi was very
        angry with Me.
        In fact, she changed her name to Mara, meaning
        "bitter." She focused so intently on the negative that
        she could not see the good plans I was working on in
        her life at that time.

Faith in Me is justified in *all* circumstances.

    Through many difficult circumstances, Naomi still was
        a woman of deep, spiritual
        understanding. Even though she did not always
        respond appropriately during her time
        of affliction, through it all she acknowledged My
        presence in her life.

You may never understand the reasons why things happen
as they do.

Even My Son, Jesus, asked, *"Why?"*

He wasn't questioning Me but expressing the deep
anguish He felt
as He took on the sins of the world. He endured for
your salvation.

Focus on the JOY in Jesus' resurrection whenever
you ask "why"!

What would I have you do now? Believe and trust that . . .

> ✍ I am faithful to meet your needs.
> ✍ You are not alone.
> ✍ I will equip you as a caregiver.
> ✍ I will change your sadness into *real* JOY. Trust Me!

I love you,
God

"For I know the plans I have for you," declares the LORD,
"plans to prosper you and not to harm you, plans to give you
hope and a future. Then you will call upon me and come and
pray to me, and I will listen to you."
—Jeremiah 29:11–12

Today, walk in the JOY of God's Word!

Read Ruth 1–4.

And at the ninth hour Jesus cried out in a loud voice,
"Eloi, Eloi, lama sabachthani?"—which means,
"My God, my God, why have you forsaken me?"
—Mark 15:34

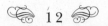

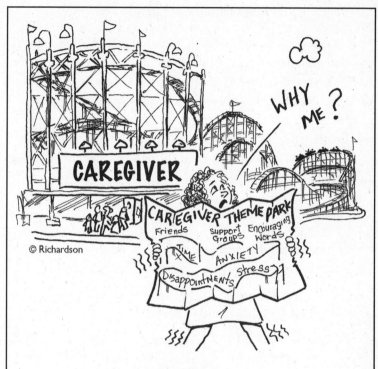

Caregiver Coaster

The Caregiver Coaster,
  emotions on the tear,
    high upon the summit,
      or valley of despair.

I'm glad that You are with me,
  Lord, keep me on the track,
    ever pressing forward,
      and never looking back.
              —*George Richardson*

Biblical Inspiration: Philippians 4:4–7

❧ Welcome to Holland ❧

As a caregiver, have you ever compared your life to a trip that you had dreamed of taking but that suddenly took you in a different direction than you planned? That's the way Emily Pearl Kingsley described her plans before she became the parent of a Down's syndrome child. Her trip closely parallels a caregiver's emotional roller coaster ride, which can be a wonderful and memorable part of our lives even though it's challenging. Here are Emily's comments:

> I am often asked to describe the experience of raising a child with a disability to try to help people who have not shared that unique experience to understand it, to imagine how it would feel. It's like this . . .
>
> When you're going to have a baby, it's like planning a fabulous vacation trip to Italy.
>
> You buy a bunch of guidebooks and make your wonderful plans—the Coliseum, Michelangelo's David, the gondolas in Venice. You may even learn some handy phrases in Italian. It's all very exciting.
>
> After months of eager anticipation, the day finally arrives. You pack your bags and off you go. Several hours later, the plane lands. The stewardess announces over the intercom, "Welcome to Holland."
>
> "Holland?" you say. "What do you mean Holland? I signed up for Italy. I'm supposed to be in Italy! All my life I've dreamed of going to Italy." But there's been a change in flight plan. They've landed in Holland, and there you must stay.
>
> The most important thing is that they haven't taken you to a horrible, disgusting, filthy place full of pestilence, famine, and disease. It's just a different

place. So you must go out and buy new guidebooks, and you must learn a whole new language. You will meet a whole new group of people that you would never have met. It's just a different place.

It's slower-paced than Italy, less flashy than Italy; but after you've been there for a while and you catch your breath, you look around and you begin to notice that Holland has windmills, tulips, and Rembrandts. But everyone you know is busy coming and going from Italy, and they're all bragging about what a wonderful time they had there. And for the rest of your life, you will say, "Yes, that's where I was supposed to go. That's what I had planned."[2]

> It's better to know and trust in the One in charge than to try to figure out "why."

The pain of unfulfilled life plans will never go away, because the loss of the dream is a very significant loss. But if you spend your life mourning the fact that you didn't get to Italy, you might never be free to feel the *real* JOY and beauty of being in Holland.

Dear Caregiver, We've asked God "why" many times, even though we believe that nothing is wasted in God's plan. Through the years we've learned that it's better to know and trust in the One in charge than to try to figure out "why."

Annetta and Karen

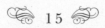

Ten Ways to be a JOYful Caregiver

C   Call for help when you need it.
A   Attitude is everything.
R   Remember you're not alone. Find a support group.
E   Educate yourself about your loved one's condition.
G   Give your best and let God do the rest.
I   Investigate options.
V   Value relationships.
E   Express your feelings; don't bury them deep inside.
R   Remember God is always with you.
S   Smile. Humor can help you through anything.

—Carmen Leal

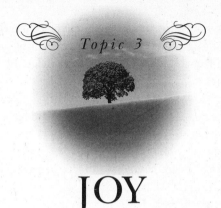

JOY

Dear God,

As I left the grocery store, the cashier said, "Have a *happy* day."

> Physically I smiled, but mentally I thought, *Happy?*
> She has no clue how many different ways I'm stretched right now as a caregiver.

Happy describes me watching the birth of my second grandchild,

> but now I'm back home and won't see him for another year. Happy?

Our single son, who lives next door, just came home from the hospital. The newest

> wrinkle in all his health problems is having seizures.
> *What do I do now?*

My husband recently had a heart stent put in and is now getting ready for gall bladder surgery.

He's been feeling miserable for so long that he's cranky.
That makes me quick-tempered. Then he gets upset,
and I start crying. I'll be so happy when he feels
better.

Finally, the cast was taken off my broken ankle, and I
couldn't wait to start therapy.
The doctor took one more MRI . . . *surprise!*
It hadn't healed, *plus* he found another hairline
fracture.
Somehow I think that I, too, am in need of a caregiver!

Lord, where's the *real* JOY in this journey?

I'm listening . . .

> *I love You,*
> *Your JOY-seeking Child*

You have made known to me the path of life; you will fill me
with joy in your presence, with eternal pleasures
at your right hand.
—Psalm 16:11

JOY

My Child,

Because you are so special to me, I know everything about
you.
> And, yes, that includes the continuous uncertainty you
> face daily as a caregiver.
> I can understand why you are asking where the *real*
> JOY is in your journey.

Real JOY is far deeper than temporary happiness that's
based on external circumstances because permanent JOY
is rooted in My presence within you.
> As you contemplate My daily presence, you will *find
> contentment in spite of circumstances.* The world can
> *never* take this *real* JOY away from you.

Take comfort that My Son, Jesus, understands what you're
going through.
> He personally knows about anger, loneliness, and the
> need for rest.
> Satan tempted Him just as he does you.

Jesus had every reason to be bitter. Yet He stayed *focused* on
His mission.
> He endured the cross, died, and rose from the grave so
> that you can have the ultimate JOY, *eternal life.*

Choosing to *trust* that I am at work in each detail of your
life will be the *sustaining* power for your soul!
> This will make a difference in your attitude and in
> your caregiving role.

JOY, a fruit of the Spirit, comes from spending time with
Me.
> Through our intimate relationship the Holy Spirit
> will draw you deeper into my *unfailing* love, and

this *real* JOY will overflow into your caregiving season.

I love you,
God

I have told you this so that my joy may be in you and that your joy may be complete.
—John 15:11

Today, walk in the JOY of God's Word!

You will fill me with joy in your presence.
—Psalm 16:11

Shout for joy, O heavens; rejoice, O earth; burst into song, O mountains! For the LORD comforts his people and will have compassion on his afflicted ones.
—Isaiah 49:13

I pray that the God who gives hope will fill you with much joy and peace while you trust in him. Then your hope will overflow by the power of the Holy Spirit.
—Romans 15:13 NCV

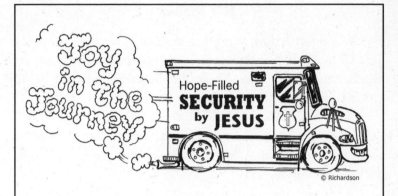

Hope-filled Security

The treasure kept in earthen jars,
   the Spirit guarantee,
      a secure and joyful ride,
         no matter what may be.

Therefore we speak,
   what we believe,
      the power of our God,
         to protect His wealth inside,
            until we leave this sod.
                —*George Richardson*

Biblical Inspiration: 2 Corinthians 4:5–18

❧ JOY Ribbon ☙

Once upon a time, a mother and daughter were shopping in a fabric store. The daughter found something she knew the mother must have. It was a bolt of ribbon with the word "JOY" printed all over it. The mother was ecstatic!

The sales attendant asked, "How much JOY do you want?"

The mother wanted to purchase the entire bolt but didn't want to seem greedy. After all, someone else might need some JOY. "I'll take five yards."

"What are you going to do with all this JOY?" asked the clerk.

Mother replied, "I'm going to save it for myself! I might not find any more JOY . . ."

Unlike the manufactured JOY ribbon, you already have an unlimited supply of God's *real* JOY. You don't have to look for JOY. God freely gives it to you.

Here are two examples of people who learned about God's JOY:

- **Moses** spent forty years in Pharaoh's house training as a prince. The next forty years he lived in exile in the wilderness as a shepherd, because he had killed an Egyptian. At age eighty, God called him to be a caregiver and deliverer of the Israelites. God was with Moses, even though at times he may have wondered where the *real* JOY was in his journey.

- **Jacquie, a caregiver in Oregon,** says, "There are some days in caregiving that you feel as if you've spent the last forty years wandering in the wilderness yourself. My husband was in so much pain, and that broke my heart. I then learned how to calm my anxious heart each morning by saying, "'This is the day the LORD has made; let us rejoice and be glad in it" (Ps. 118:24).

Thank you, Lord, for the gift of today.' I then looked at the day through different eyes because I looked for His blessings."

Caregiving is a difficult journey, but oh the JOY that fills your heart as you learn to *trust* in God's *faithfulness*! Trust comes from knowing Him. You get to know Him better as you spend time in His Word. Now that's a JOY-filled relationship!

Oh, the JOY that fills your heart as you learn to trust in God's *faithfulness*!

Dear Caregiver, When we were caregivers, it was difficult to always see His presence because we were so caught up in our duties. No, we weren't always happy, but it was the true JOY of God's presence that sustained us. How do you feel God's presence in the caregiving challenges you are facing right now? We'd love to know! Contact us at joy4caringhearts@gmail.com and share your story! You might read your story in *Nuggets of Hope,* a newsletter for caregivers.

Annetta and Karen

Two caregivers face similar struggles. One is destroyed and thinks, *I'll never get over this.* The other is despondent but determined and says, *God will get me through this!* Our knowledge of God's Word affects our attitude every single day.

—Author Unknown

Attitude

Dear God,

I'm having "a terrible, horrible, no good, very bad day"![13]

I planned to pick Grandpa up early so we wouldn't be late
for the new doctor's appointment.
Just as I was walking out the door the phone rang.
"Mom, I forgot my lunch. Can you drop it off?"
"No problem!"

Grandpa needed to begin his new medication today, so we
stopped at the pharmacy.
He forgot his cash, and I didn't have my credit card
with me.
We have to make another trip.
No problem!

Just as I brought him home and thought I'd quickly mow
his grass, he had a bowel problem.
That's so embarrassing for him; and it's *no* picnic for
me either!

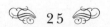

Immediately I had a choice to make—an attitude choice!
My mood would not only affect him, but also it could
affect my family's mood.
Was it really worth the cost of getting upset?

I may not be able to choose if I will be sick or healthy
or if my loved one will have a good day or not,
but I can *choose* my attitude.

Help me, Lord! I'm trying to remain calm, but my tears
keep coming.

I'm listening . . .

I love You,
Your Stressed-Out Child

Your attitude should be the same as that of Christ Jesus . . .
—Philippians 2:5

My Child,

It's okay to let your stress out through tears. I understand,
and other caregivers can relate, too.

You know what those days are like when you are grateful
and feel privileged to be a caregiver.
> And you know about the days filled with unexpected
> frustrations.
> I know you do your best. I've seen the admirable job
> you are doing.

I also know the anxiety you experience
because of those endless details
> and undesirable situations.
> Even then, on those days that are
> so terrible and horrible, never
> doubt that
> through My strength you can do
> this.

Find comfort in
My Word.

My dear child, listen, and find comfort in My Word:

> But he said to me, "My grace is sufficient for you, for
> my power is made perfect in weakness." Therefore I
> will boast all the more gladly of my weaknesses, so
> that the power of Christ may rest upon me. For the
> sake of Christ, then, I am content with weaknesses,
> insults, hardships, persecutions, and calamities. For
> when I am weak, then I am strong.
>
> —2 Corinthians 12:9–10 ESV

I am a God of personal details.
> St. Paul, one of My servants, experienced shipwrecks,
> beatings, and imprisonments.
> Yet *he refused to give up*! His key to surviving, in spite
> of the circumstances,

was being content because he knew My faithfulness
and trusted that I am in control.

The *real* JOY you have from My presence will always be
your strength.

Focus on this, and it will transform your mind and
attitude into Christ's likeness.

My precious child, *you are not alone*!

I love you,
God

*I know what it is to be in need, and I know what it is to have
plenty. I have learned the secret of being content in any
and every situation, whether well fed or hungry, whether
living in plenty or in want. I can do everything
through him who gives me strength.*
—Philippians 4:12–13

Today, walk in the JOY of God's Word!

Depend on the LORD; trust him, and he will take care of you.
—Psalm 37:5 NCV

*He guides the humble in what is right and teaches them his
way. All the ways of the Lord are loving and faithful for those
who keep the demands of his covenant.*
—Psalm 25:9–10

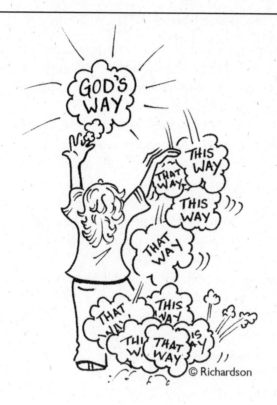

I've Learned

I've learned to brush aside the thoughts,
    that throw me off the course,
an attitude created new,
    all holy, right, and true,
where Jesus is the source.

—George Richardson

Biblical Inspiration: Ephesians 4:20–24

❧ Three Hairs—A New Attitude ❧

There once was a woman who woke up one morning, looked in the mirror, and noticed she only had three hairs on her head. "Well," she said, "I think I'll braid my hair today." So she did, and she had a wonderful day.

The next day, she woke up, looked in the mirror, and saw that she had only two hairs on her head. "Hmm," she said, "I think I'll part my hair down the middle today." So she did, and she had a grand day.

The next day she woke up, looked in the mirror, and noticed that she had only one hair on her head. "Well," she said, "today I'm going to wear my hair in a pony tail." So she did, and she had a fun, fun day.

The next day she woke up, looked in the mirror, and noticed that there wasn't a single hair on her head. "Yea!" she exclaimed. "I don't have to fix my hair today!"[4]

If only all of us could have the same attitude—to look at the blessings and not the burdens. Satan knows our lack of contentment that lends itself to a poor attitude. He will attack our areas of weakness every time.

> Look at the blessings and not the burdens.

Eve was vulnerable to Satan's line of attack. How could she be happy when she wasn't allowed to eat from one of the fruit trees? Eve was willing to accept Satan's insinuations without checking with God. She fell for the idea that the one item that was not within her reach would make her happy.

Sound familiar? As her descendants, we open ourselves to envy, greed, jealousy, worry, and all kinds of selfish behavior in order to satisfy our longings. And when we follow through on our impulses, the satisfaction we find is hollow and quickly vanishes.

God has given us all we need to be happy. But the *real* JOY comes in knowing that God loves us so much that He gave His "one and only Son that whoever believes in him shall not perish but have eternal life" (John 3:16). Now that's contentment that will put us on the right track, the track to a great attitude!

Dear Caregiver, Whether you realize it or not, your kind words are an encouragement to those who need care. Love generously, care deeply, speak kindly, and leave the rest to God. Life isn't about waiting for the storm to pass; it's about learning to dance in the rain! Attitude is everything. Have a JOY-filled day!

Annetta and Karen

Mary's choice to sit at Jesus' feet was not made out of obligation but devotion. Which do you have? It makes a difference in how you react or respond to your overwhelming day.

—Author Unknown

Overwhelmed

Dear God,

Today I am absolutely *overwhelmed*! I'm trying to . . .

- keep up with the yard work.
- prepare job resumes to find work after being let go after fifteen years.
- work a part-time job.
- get my father to his daily radiation treatments and weekly blood tests.
- keep one step ahead in paying the monthly bills.

I'm also overwhelmed by other demands that I cannot meet and decisions that I just cannot face.

I'm tired, Father. I'm really, really tired of trying to keep one step ahead in life!
I keep looking forward to the day when . . . life slows down . . . all my problems are solved (yeah, right!) . . . and I can know what contentment really means!

How could Paul talk about being content with all the
problems he had to face?
Wasn't he ever overwhelmed?

Lord, I desperately need You to refresh my weary spirit and
give me a fresh perspective today,
but I'm having trouble finding time even to talk to
You.

I'm listening . . .

I love You,
Your Overwhelmed Child

Cast your cares on the LORD and he will sustain you; he will
never let the righteous fall.
—Psalm 55:22

Overwhelmed

My Child,

Sometimes living just takes the life out of you, doesn't it?
    I understand why you, as a frazzled caregiver, are
        longing for contentment.

Making the time to take care of yourself—getting rest,
    exercising, and eating properly—
        is not only preventative maintenance, but also it can be
        a time of contentment.
        A calm within you can also be felt when you listen to
        music, read, or
        do number puzzles while waiting at appointments.
        However, these are
            temporary.

The foundation to *lasting*
    inner peace is found only
    in one source, My Son,
    Jesus Christ.
        Just as you enjoy doing
        different things with
        your friends, enJOY
        your time with Me.

> My presence is your contentment, even in your most frazzled and frantic moments.

    - Be spontaneous in the way you worship Me.
    - Express your love through whistling a hymn.
    - When you go for a walk, enjoy the smell of
      freshly mown grass.
    - Write Me a letter, and let your thoughts flow.

I love you, My child. That's why I am *your* caregiver!
    I long for you to spend time in My presence, listening
      to My voice,
    even in the middle of the things that overwhelm you.
    My presence is your contentment, even in your most
    frazzled and frantic moments.

St. Paul knew the secret of being content, even in the worst
circumstances.
He continually had trials that overwhelmed him, but
he knew he was connected to Me,
his ultimate source of strength.
He drew close to Me and was content!

Take life one day at a time. EnJOY our relationship.

I love you,
God

Draw near to God, and he will draw near to you . . .
—James 4:8 ESV

Today, walk in the JOY of God's Word!

I am not saying this because I am in need, for I have learned
to be content whatever the circumstances.
—Philippians 4:11

Come with me by yourselves to a quiet place and get some rest.
—Mark 6:31

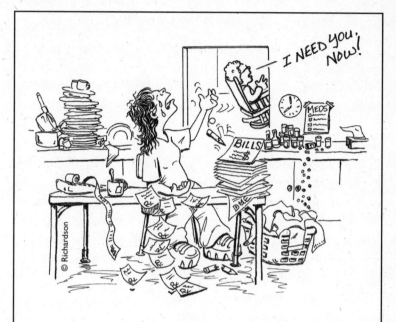

Overcome

God will help me trust His grace,
    when overcome with tears,
For in my weakness comes His strength,
    proven through the years.
—*George Richardson*

Biblical Inspiration: Psalm 142:7

🍃 This Is the Day 🍃

Once upon a time, a preacher went to conduct a series of meetings quite far from his home, so he was invited to stay overnight with one of the church families. When he woke up in the morning, he saw the words scratched on the bedroom window pane, "This is the day." He had never seen anything like this before, so he asked his hostess, "What does this mean?"

She explained that for many years she had been a Christian. However, her life had been filled with worry, and she knew little happiness and felt no JOY. She kept living in the future, hoping for a better day, but it never came. She would think that maybe when the children grew up, possibly when the mortgage was paid off, or perhaps when things weren't so busy, then that inner peace would come to her.

Then one morning, while she was having devotions, she read, "This is the day the LORD has made, let us rejoice and be glad in it" (Ps. 118:24). Like a shining light from heaven above, those words illuminated her heart and mind.

This very day was a gift from God.

She had always anticipated contentment in Christ but never had known it. For the first time she realized that God's marvelous contentment was to be claimed in all things that overwhelmed her. She realized that the *present* was for her, and the *future* belongs to God.

As a lasting reminder, she scratched the words on the window pane. Every morning thereafter, when she woke up, she read, "This is the day . . ." not tomorrow, not next week, not next year, but this very day was a gift from God to her.

Dear Caregiver, Has that ever happened to you when reading Scripture? It's like God pulls out His heavenly highlighter and circles a verse just for that moment! He will be your help and guide in all that you do during this season of your life. Write this on a piece of paper and keep it with you at all times:

> *Dear Caregiver,*
>
> *Don't worry about a thing!*
>
> *I will be handling all your problems today.*
>
> *Love,*
> *GOD*

Annetta and Karen

Role Reversal
So many years you have been there
To love and cherish, honor, care.
But now it's time to lean on me.
Lord, help me be just what he needs.

—Dr. Vicki L. Gilliam

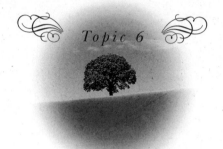

Tough Love

Dear God,

It seems like yesterday that Dad was teaching me how to
drive!
> He worried that I would hit someone
> or pull out in front of a car
> or lose control by over-correcting
> or, even worse, get a ticket and lose my license!

Now the role is reversed, and I'm in a tough love zone.
> I worry about the very same situations he drilled into
> me.
> It's so hard to love someone, want him to be safe,
> and yet help him to feel independent.

How am I going to tell him in a positive way so that I
won't hurt him
> . . . won't make him feel worthless
> . . . won't make him feel guilty that I'm driving him
> everywhere?
> His car keys are his independence!

Oh, Lord, I feel so inadequate to implement this tough
 love.
     Give me wisdom to know the right time to tell him.
     Give me strength not to let him talk me out of this.
     Help me to meet the challenges in my caregiving.

I'm listening . . .

> *I love You,*
> *Your Child Who Needs Courage*

> *On the day I called, you answered me;*
> *my strength of soul you increased.*
> *—Psalm 138:3*

Tough Love

My Child,

I am so glad you came to Me with your concerns.
    I am your strength and your stronghold.
    The JOY of My presence will always be your refuge.

A loving relationship is one to cherish.
    Your father had the same feelings about you when he
       had to use tough love.
    Now it's your turn.

Do you remember when you wanted to stay late at the
    homecoming dance?
    You weren't happy about not being given permission to
       do so,
    but you didn't love your father any less for it.

I didn't allow Moses to walk into the Promised Land,
    but he didn't love Me any less.

And remember when My only Son asked that "this cup" be
    taken from Him?
    He still loved Me through all the suffering and pain.

In the story that Jesus told about the prodigal son and how
    he squandered his inheritance,
       the young man returned to his father with a humble
         and repentant heart.
       His father still loved him dearly and ran to meet him
         when he saw him coming down the road. He even
         organized a feast in his son's honor.

Yes, my child, it's very tough love,
    but remember how much I care for you.
    I will be with you *always*.

I love you,
God

For the LORD is good and His love endures forever;
His faithfulness continues through all generations.
—Psalm 100:5

Today, walk in the JOY of God's Word!

Read about the prodigal son in Luke 15:11–32.

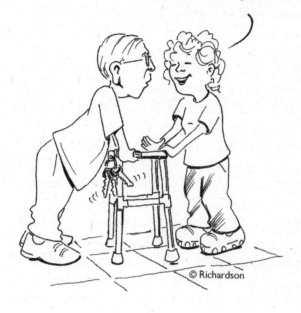

Tough Love

Let me speak the truth in love,
    your cherished key is safe above,
kept by Jesus—one day you'll soar,
    but while on earth, you'll drive no more.
—*George Richardson*

Biblical Inspiration: Proverbs 24:26

Three Frogs on a Log

A young boy approached his father and said, "Dad, there are three frogs on a log close to a lake. One of them decided to jump in. How many remain on the log?"

"Hmmm, well, let me see," said his father. "Three frogs, one decided to jump. That leaves two."

"No, Dad, all three of them remained in the same place."

"But how? You said that one decided to jump. Then there are only two left!"

"Yes, Dad, that's what I said. One of them *decided* to jump. It doesn't mean that he *did* jump."

Sometimes we decide, plan, and visualize what we want to do. We can even see the JOY of accomplishing the goal. Often, we are just like the frog. We decide to do something, but we don't put our thoughts or words into action.

With God, though, things are different. He decided to love and save mankind, but His decision also became an *action.* He sent His Son to take our sins upon Himself and suffer our punishment. This is how His love was put into action—through His sacrifice. That was tough love. And look at the *real* JOY that action has brought us!

We can decide what should be done and talk about it, but if we don't put the "talk" into action, no good can come from it. It's just words in the air. Don't let words be just words. Let your decisions become actions.

Dear Caregiver, From experience, we know that there will be tough decisions as the roles are reversed because your loved one is no longer looking out for him or herself. Remember, it's for his or her own safety.

Annetta and Karen

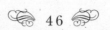

Living with Parent

Dear God,

We've made a decision to bring Mom into our home so
    that we can provide the care she needs,
        but there are so many questions that come to my mind
           that
        I can barely think of anything else.

I'm scared!

Will we ever have time for ourselves?
        Would it be okay to have Mom go to an adult daycare
           one day a week?
        Can we afford all the expenses that will add up because
           of this decision?

I look back on all the love and care that she has given to
    my family and me,
        and I wouldn't even consider not caring for her.
        But now I have to face the situation head-on, and
        my mind is racing with all the "what if's" and questions:

- What if the grandchildren make too much noise when they visit?
- What if she doesn't like the friends my college-aged son brings home?
- What if she interferes with decisions my husband and I have made?
- Should I have her try to do things around the house? Or would that be asking too much of her?

I'm scared, God!

I'm listening . . .

> *I love You,*
> *Your Nervous Child*

Cast your cares on the LORD and he will sustain you;
he will never let the righteous fall.
—Psalm 55:22

Living with Parent

My Child,

I have said, "Come to me, all who are heavy-laden, and I
   will give you rest." I have endless
      strength for your days ahead so that you can face your
      questions and future challenges.

Showing respect to older generations teaches young people
   how to respect and treat older adults,
      including you. Don't set older adults aside and lead them
      to believe that their lives and opinions don't count.

Open communication is always best. Talk with your
   mother about any concerns you have about
      expenses and how she feels about an "activity day" out
      with other seniors.

The older generation needs to feel
   wanted, useful, loved, and appreciated.

They also want to feel that they are significant in the lives
   of other people,
      especially family and friends.
      Gray hair or a bent body doesn't mean that they are
         any different on the inside.
      They still have feelings.

Cherish your mother's wit and wisdom, and be thankful
   that you can enjoy your time together.
      This helps her feel worthwhile.
      Families are gifts from Me and are to be loved and
         nurtured.

As I watched My Son on the cross, I remember how He
   looked at His mother and the disciple
      whom He loved. He said to His mother, "Woman,
         behold your son!"

Next He said to the disciple, "Behold, your mother!"
From that hour on the disciple took her to his own
    home (John 19:26–27).
Think of the pain that Jesus was in, yet He looked
    down from the cross, saw His mother,
and was concerned about what would happen to her.

It's not always possible for your loved one to stay in your
    home, but if it is,
    the JOYS can be numerous. I promise you *strength* to
    get through each day, *comfort* for the tears, and a
    Light for the way.

I love you,
God

The mouth of the righteous man utters wisdom,
and his tongue speaks what is just.
—Psalm 37:30

Today, walk in the JOY of God's Word!

Come to me, all you who are weary and burdened,
and I will give you rest.
—Matthew 11:28

They will still bear fruit in old age,
they will stay fresh and green . . .
—Psalm 92:14

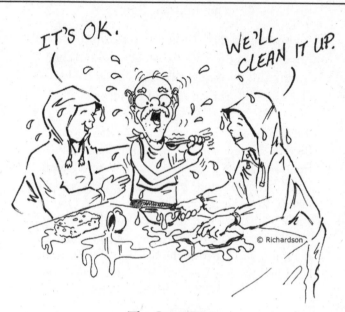

The Soup Line

Some days it is a challenge,
   to really keep it neat,
      as soup slides down my collar,
      and peas are on my seat.

For you it is an honor,
   repaying all you've done,
      teaching table manners,
      when we were having fun.

And now the role's reversing,
   but we will never fuss,
      'cause playing in our food,
      was always fun for us.

                   —*George Richardson*

Biblical Inspiration: Deuteronomy 5:16

❧ The Wooden Bowl ❧

Do you love fairy tales? The Brothers Grimm compiled over two hundred tales in the 1800s that were told to them through oral tradition. This particular tale dates as far back as 1535 and was titled, "The Old Man and His Grandson":

> There was once a very old man whose eyes had become dim, his ears dull of hearing, and his knees trembled. When he sat at the table he could hardly hold the spoon and spilled the broth upon the tablecloth or let it run out of his mouth. His son and his son's wife were disgusted by this, so the old grandfather at last had to sit in the corner behind the stove. They gave him his food in an earthenware bowl and not even enough of it. He would look towards the family table with his eyes full of tears.

> One day his trembling hands couldn't hold the bowl, and it fell to the ground and broke. The young wife scolded him, but he said nothing and only sighed. Then they bought him a wooden bowl for a few pennies, out of which he had to eat.

> On another day they were sitting like this when the little grandson of four years old began to gather together some bits of wood upon the ground. "What are you doing there?" asked the father.

> "I am making a little trough," answered the child, "for Father and Mother to eat out of when I am big."

> The man and his wife looked at each other for a while and began to cry. Then they took the old grandfather to the table and henceforth always let him eat with them, and likewise said nothing if he did spill a little of anything.

Dear Caregiver, Live-in parents are likely to be more demanding than infants, more exhausting than toddlers, and more unpredictable and moody than teens. There will be days when you question the wisdom of your decision. But God is faithful. He will give you strength for as long as having your live-in parent is the best alternative.

Annetta and Karen

Self-care is never a selfish act—it is simply good stewardship of the only gift I have, the gift I was put on earth to offer to others. Anytime we can listen to true self, and give it the care it requires, we do so not only for ourselves, but for the many others whose lives we touch.

—Parker Palmer

Personal Health

Dear God,

I knew my friend really meant it when she looked me in
the eyes, shook her finger, and said,
*"You need to start taking care of yourself,
or you won't be able to take care of your child!"*

What she didn't know was that the minute she left, I burst
into tears.
She had no clue how I'm struggling with my own
health.
My fibromyalgia is getting worse and so is my weight!
I don't know if the pain in my chest is real or if it's just
anxiety.

I feel so guilty thinking about *my* health when it's my son
who needs the care!
I keep telling myself, *If I don't feel better tomorrow, I'll
call the doctor.*
Tomorrow hasn't come yet.

My son needs me now. I'm still trying to learn how to
    manage the infusion tube
        and not jump out of my
            skin when the monitor's
            alarm goes off.

I'm at a crossroad in my life,
    Lord. Which way do I go?
        I'm wise enough to know
           that he needs an alert and
           healthy mom.
        But how do I do all of this?

*I'm at a crossroad in
my life, Lord. Which
way do I go?*

I'm listening . . .

                I love You,
                Your Health-Deprived Child

The Lord rescues me when He sees that my strength is gone.
He has mercy on me when He sees how helpless I am.
        —Deuteronomy 32:36 GNT

Personal Health

My Child,

I understand how much you want to be a dedicated caregiver,
> but I also know how you are sacrificing your own health to do so.
> Remember that taking care of yourself will affect *everyone* else in your life!

Eating right, sleeping, exercising, and relaxing are vital.
> Ignoring any of these can make you tense, irritable, and unable to tackle even little things. The longer your body goes unattended, the more your body, emotions, and mind will suffer.

It's difficult to balance the needs of those you care for plus take care of your own well-being.
> While it may seem selfish to find care for your son while you do something for yourself,
> it doesn't mean you are weak but *very wise*!

Taking care of yourself involves getting rest for your body, renewal for your mind,
> and nurture for your spirit.
> Maintaining your mental, physical, and spiritual health is critical to your well-being! Good health is a *choice* you must make, not a pill you can take.

You have many friends who have offered to stay with him.
Accept their offers.
> It's their way of showing you they care about your family.
> Make the time to go for a complete physical and a mammogram.
> Encourage your husband to have his physical and prostate check also.

Your son loves to look at the picture by his bed. He has almost memorized the verse:
> "He gives strength to the weary and increases the
> power of the weak.
> Even youths grow tired and weary, and young men
> stumble and fall;
> but those who hope in the LORD will renew their
> strength.
> They will soar on wings like eagles; they will run and
> not grow weary,
> they will walk and not be faint" (Isa. 40:29–31).

Even the strongest people get tired at times, but My power and strength *never* diminish.
> The JOY of My presence will be your source of
> strength throughout this stressful season.
> Caregiving is not just a two-person, but a three-person
> relationship—
> your loved one . . . you . . . and Me!

I love you,
God

Dear friend, I pray that you may enjoy good health
and that all may go well with you even as your soul is
getting along well.
—3 John 1:2

Today, walk in the JOY of God's Word!

Why are you downcast, O my soul? Why so disturbed within
me? Put your hope in God, for I will yet praise him,
my Savior and my God.
—Psalm 43:5

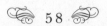

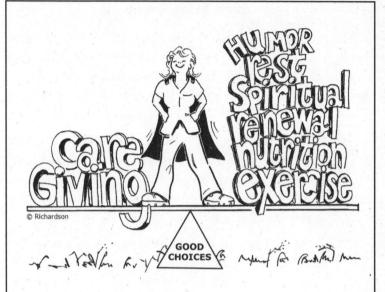

Good Choices

Balancing, balancing,
    what an act,
        what grace, what form, what flow.

The care you give,
    equals your take,
        good choices in the know.
                —*George Richardson*

Biblical Inspiration: Proverbs 14:1

❧ Stress Management ☙

Major life changes, such as caregiving, always become stressors because they force us to adapt to new situations. You can't avoid stress, but there are ways to manage it. Try some of these tips to help you become stress-resistant. It's a choice you can make.

- **Change the way you look at things**. How you view challenges may be more stressful than the actual situation. Sort out problems—which are real and which are simply imagined? Deal with them as they are and not as you think they are.

- **Accept what you cannot change.** Change what you can. But if you can't change it, learn to live with it. Tomorrow will still come!

- **Focus on concerns, not worries**. A concern can be changed, such as setting an alarm clock when you're concerned about getting up on time. A worry is something you can't do anything about. Give it to God. He's waiting!

- **Deal with one problem at a time.** Sort out your priorities and deal with them in the order of their importance.

- **Be flexible**. Give in occasionally. If you do, others will, too.

- **Get enough rest, relaxation, and sleep. Eat healthy.** Give your body a chance to recover from day to day.

- **Work off stress.** Go for a walk. Take deep breaths and exhale slowly while you count to ten.

- **Talk to someone**. Talking, instead of eating, often gives you a different perspective. A burden shared is much less of a burden.

- **Read God's Word daily. Pray.** God has a way of turning things around for you. Don't miss out on a blessing because it isn't packaged in the way that you expect!

Dear Caregiver, In this book, under the topic of Physical Fitness, there are more excellent tips. We call them JOYercise. Caregivers love them! We hope you will, too.

Annetta and Karen

Since He took care of our greatest need at Calvary by giving us Christ, then you, [dear caregiver], can be sure God will take care of everything else He considers important to us.

—Charles Swindoll

Trust

Dear God,

Circumstances are out of control and so am I. Help!

I am frustrated!
> The agency has now sent out three different people to
> assess her care.
> One says she needs therapy to strengthen her leg, while
> the next one disagrees.
> The third said she'll get back to me.
> I'm still waiting! Whom can I trust?

I am worried.
> She always did her own shots before, and now she's
> putting her trust in me.

I am embarrassed.
> The neighbors say it is not a bother to stay while I
> make another quick trip to get something she needs,
> but I just can't ask them any more.

Her personality is changing, and it makes them
uncomfortable.
I just don't know what to do!

My son doesn't have time to
come mow the yard. The
grandchildren have called
again
begging me to come to their
musical.

There is just one giant
obstacle after another
in my life.

There is just one giant obstacle
after another in my life. Is it
any wonder that I went to the
workshop and tried to make a bird house, but I
hammered so hard I splintered the wood?

There's so much going on in my life.
Changes. Challenges. Choices.
Right now life looks hopeless. Help!

I'm listening . . .

I love You
Your Hopeless Child

For those who know your name will trust in you, for you,
LORD, have never forsaken those who seek you.
—Psalm 9:10

Trust

My Child,

Trust Me. After all, David killed a giant with a single stone.
　　While others thought the situation was hopeless and
　　　　the giant was too big to hit,
　　　　David had a different perspective . . . Goliath was too
　　　　big to miss!

To see your circumstances with human eyes is to see a
　　hopeless end. But to look
　　　　at your Goliath-sized obstacles through the grace-filled
　　　　eyes of My Son, Jesus Christ, you will find *endless*
　　　　hope. I promise!

My promises do not mean that if you trust in Me, you will
　　escape the disappointments,
　　　　discouragement, and doubts that are all a part of your
　　　　caregiving journey.
　　　　They do, however, guarantee that I will *never leave you,*
　　　　no matter what you face!
　　　　Trust in My faithfulness.

To slay your giant concern about being closer to her at
　　night, talk to your children about your options. The
　　neighbors offered to help mow.
　　　　This will allow them to show how much they care for
　　　　you in their own unique way.

Satan works hard to complicate your life so he can steal
　　your JOY.
　　　　Whenever he does, refocus on those who trusted Me,
　　　　such as
　　　　Daniel in the lion's den;
　　　　Noah, who built the ark when he had not seen rain;
　　　　and
　　　　Shadrach, Meshach, and Abednego in the furnace.

I love to have you read My Word so that your trust will grow deeper and your faith stronger.
You'll see my faithfulness everywhere, and your heart will be elevated from daily distractions to lasting confidence.

When things become difficult, look to Me for strength.

Trust Me. Trust My Word. And when things become difficult, look to Me for strength.
Seek my face always, and I will be there for you.

I love you,
God

Trust in him at all times, O people; pour out your hearts to him, for God is our refuge.
—Psalm 62:8

Today, walk in the JOY of God's Word!

Read about Daniel in the lion's den in Daniel 6:1–28.
Read about Noah and the ark in Genesis 6:9–9:17.
Read about Shadrach, Meshach, and Abednego in Daniel 2:49–3:30.

The LORD is faithful to all his promises
and loving toward all he has made.
—Psalm 143:13

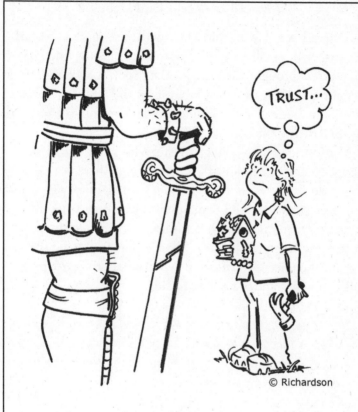

© Richardson

Trust

I will succeed I trust,
    with giants it's a must.
I have no skill to hammer home,
    a fortress strong to brace.
I must rely upon my God,
    that He'll supply the grace.
          —*George Richardson*

Biblical Inspiration: Hebrews 4:14–16

❧ Forced to Accept Paid Debt ❧

A friend was having breakfast with his son one Saturday morning at a small café. As they were finishing their meal, the waitress brought their check, then took it away, and then brought it back again. She placed it on the table, smiled, and said, "Somebody in the restaurant paid for your meal. You're all set." She then walked away.

As my friend was telling the story he said, "I had such a strange feeling of helplessness as I sat there. There was nothing I could do. It had been taken care of. To insist on paying would have been pointless. All I could do was trust that what she said was actually true and then live with that—which meant getting up and leaving the restaurant. My acceptance of what she said gave me a choice: to live like it was true or to create my own reality in which the bill was not paid."

This is our invitation to trust that: we don't owe anything, something is already true about us, something has already been done, and something has been there all along. This is our invitation to trust that grace pays the bill.

The following is a true story: A woman broke her arm and had to depend on her husband to shave her armpit. Well, he had shaved his face for years, so what was the problem? He certainly had years of experience and knew how to shave, didn't he? The problem was one of trust. Total dependence on another doesn't come easily for us, but isn't that what God wants us to do? To put our total dependence in Him?[5]

On the surface, trusting that someone will care for us seems legitimate; however, it truly deepens our trust level when we have to trust that no harm or pain will come to us from another.

In Paul's second letter to the Corinthians (1:8–10), Paul explains how he and Timothy endured such terrible hardships and suffering in Asia that they thought they were going to die. However, they felt this happened because they then had to trust in God and not in themselves, knowing that God is the true Comforter and Deliverer.

We often depend on our own skills and abilities when life seems easy, but we turn to God when we feel unable to help ourselves. Depending on God is realizing that we are powerless without Him and that we need His constant touch in our lives. God is our source of power, and we can put our complete trust in Him for all our needs.

Dear Caregiver, Think of a blessing that begins with each of the letters in the word "trust." (We did the first letter for you.) Praise the Lord who is our strength, our guide, and our hope.

T . . . Telephone call from friends

R . . .

U . . .

S . . .

T . . .

Karen and Annetta

An encouraging word or simply a positive attitude can make the difference to someone who's given up hope!

—Barbara Johnson

Making a Difference

Dear God,

Today was one of those days when nothing went as
   planned.
       We got up early because the home health nurse was
          coming.
       As for the rest of the morning, if something could go
          wrong, it did!
       I was having my own little pity party. *I needed a break!*

Then, in the midst of all that was happening, a friend "just
   happened" to call.
       Although I'd never gone, she encouraged me to go
          with her to her support group meeting.
       I'm so glad I went. Why didn't I do it sooner?

Even though our situations varied, we had much in
   common.
       We cried! It's difficult to see our loved ones hurting.
       We laughed! That was so healing.
       We prayed! How comforting!
       We hugged! I felt accepted and loved.

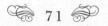

The meeting really made a difference in my life. It gave me
a new perspective:

      ✍ That being kind is more important than being
        right.

      ✍ That the Lord didn't do it all in one day.
        (What makes me think I can?)

      ✍ That I can't choose how I feel, but I can
        choose what I do about it.[6]

I can't wait to go back. Their encouragement energized my
spirit.

    But Lord, I'm feeling guilty because I really enjoyed
      myself tonight.

    Is it okay to feel this way?

I'm listening . . .

I love You,
Your Grateful Child

Let us not give up meeting together, as some are in the habit of
doing, but let us encourage one another . . .
—Hebrews 10:25

Making a Difference

My Child,

I take such delight in you, and that's why I'm smiling!
 It's so good to see you encouraged and refreshed.
 And whether you realize it or not, *you* also made a
  difference in their lives.
 Without even realizing it, you naturally encourage
  others.

Don't feel guilty about taking time for yourself. These
 mini-breaks are not a luxury.
 They are absolutely necessary. Self-care is an essential
  part of caregiving.
 You can give more freely and effectively when you've
  replenished yourself!

Caregiving can be a rewarding and a life-affirming experience.
 It can also be draining and exhausting.
 Never be embarrassed to ask for help or to get respite
  from support groups.
 This will help to restore your vitality and you will
  discover your wellspring of loving care.
 Everyone benefits!

Being a caregiver means caring for yourself as well!

When Moses was caring for the Israelites, leading My
 people from Egypt to their homeland,
 he was overwhelmed with his responsibilities.
 Jethro, his father-in-law, expressed concern that Moses
  was going to wear himself out
 and that he could not handle the burden all by himself.
 Moses accepted the life-changing advice and found
  others to help carry the load.

Moses' contentment, even in trials, came from his intimate
 relationship with Me.

In his own unique way, he was *making a difference* as
he cared for others.

Come often, just like Moses did, and sit at My feet. You
will be strengthened
from the JOY of My presence!

I know that, just as Moses did, you have made personal
sacrifices that people around you do not
always understand, acknowledge, or appreciate. So
meditate on this thought—to the world, you might
be only one person; but to one person, you just
might be the world!

Caregiver, you are a *silent hero*, making a difference because
of the *real* JOY
of Jesus Christ, who lives within you!

I love you,
God

But I have raised you up for this very purpose, that I might
show you my power and that my name might be proclaimed
in all the earth.
—Exodus 9:16

Today, walk in the JOY of God's Word!

Read about Jethro and Moses in Exodus 18:13–27.

Your love has given me great joy and encouragement, because
you, brother, have refreshed the hearts of the saints.
—Philemon 1:7

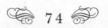

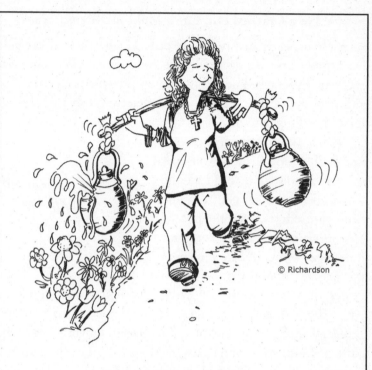

© Richardson

The Difference Flows

Spirit-filled I need to be,
      for Your love to flow.
The parched to find a mountain lake,
      the chilled a quilt in winter's blow.
So my silent difference makes,
      my Father's love to show.
              —*George Richardson*

Biblical Inspiration: John 7:38–39

❦ I'm a Cracked Pot. Can I Make a Difference? ❦

A water bearer had two large pots which hung on the pole he carried across his neck. One pot was perfect. The other was cracked. The cracked pot was ashamed of its own imperfections and miserable that it was only able to accomplish half of what it had been made to do.

"I'm a bitter failure. I always lose half of my load. Because of my flaws, you have to do all the work, and you don't get full value from your efforts," said the pot.

As a caregiver, *you are making a difference*!

The water bearer felt sorry for the cracked pot. "As we return to the master's house, I want you to notice there are beautiful flowers only along one side of the path. That's because I have always known about your flaw, and I took advantage of it. I planted flower seeds on your side of the path, and every day, while we walked back from the stream, you have watered them. Because of your flaw, I've been able to pick flowers to decorate my master's table. Without you, just the way you are, he wouldn't have had this beauty to grace his table."

There is nothing insignificant that you do in Christ's name that goes unnoticed by the Lord. Never doubt that as a caregiver, *you are making a difference*!

Dear Caregiver, Encouragement comes in many different ways, including the permission to feel what you feel. Ask God to guide you to make a difference because you understand what it means to be a caregiver. Don't forget to remind others that He is their caregiver, too!

Annetta and Karen

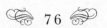

Time for Me

Dear God,

I'm at the end of my rope.
   I really, really need some time for me, even though this
      little voice keeps whispering,
   "You should be able to do it all! Just try harder!"

A year ago I had two fully capable parents. Now they need
   me at their house most of the time.
      Whenever I bring up alternative living arrangements,
         they get stubborn.
      Add to that stress that I have a teenaged daughter who
         is bipolar and learning to drive.

I quit my job, thinking it would help, but I'm still grumpy
   and snap at everyone—
      including the paper boy. I'm no fun anymore. In fact, *I*
         don't even like me!

I love my family. I'm constantly thinking about how I can
   be the perfect caregiver, and

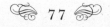

yet I keep wanting some time just for me. I'm ashamed to admit it, but I'd love to

. . . relax in the shower instead of washing and running!

. . . go to bed and sleep without waiting on the phone to ring!

. . . have a massage at a spa.

Lord, how can I survive?

I'm listening . . .

> *I love You,*
> *Your Grumpy Child*

Then, because so many people were coming and going that they did not even have a chance to eat, he said to them, "Come with me by yourselves to a quiet place and get some rest."
—Mark 6:31

My Child,

It's difficult to balance caring for older parents and a family member
> and meeting everyone's individual needs.
>> There's no time left for you
>>> to replenish yourself.
>> Everyone has their limits as
>>> a caregiver.
>> Knowing your limits will
>>> help to prevent burnout.

Knowing your limits will help to prevent burnout.

When Jesus asked His disciples
> to follow Him, they, like you,
> experienced a new lifestyle.
>> In their own way they, too,
>>> were caregivers meeting multiple needs of others.
>> They didn't always find it easy to consider their own health.
>> So Jesus said, "Come with me by yourselves to a *quiet place*
>> and get some rest" (Mark 6:31).
>> Jesus knew that if they were to be *effective*, they needed periodic rest and renewal.

You mentioned a massage at the spa. That would help you
> to relax temporarily.
>> But I also invite you to come to a spa for your *soul*.
>> It will give you everlasting hope and *real* JOY from My presence.
>> As you read My Word, you'll find restoration and peace unlike the world offers.

My spa for the soul is a place of solitude, a time just for *you* and Me . . .

- where silence will slow you down and refresh your thirsty soul.
- where I will massage your heart with My grace.
- where obedience will become a matter of love rather than obligation.
- where inward solitude will have outward expressions.

My dearest child, soul-nurturing is not a luxury, and it is not optional; it is a necessity.

I am waiting to restore your soul. Come.

I love you,
God

Be still, and know that I am God . . .
—Psalm 46:10

Today, walk in the JOY of God's Word!

Read about Jesus calling the disciples in Matthew 4:18–22.

And the peace of God, which transcends all understanding, will guard your hearts and your minds in Christ Jesus.
—Philippians 4:7

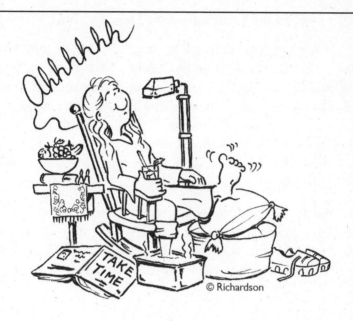

© Richardson

Time For Me

A quiet place,
    to get some rest,
        "Come with me," He said.

But when they docked,
    the need was there,
        to provide the folks with care.

With Him their rest,
    was in the boat,
        while mine is in the chair.
                —*George Richardson*

Biblical Inspiration: Mark 6:31

🌿 Spa for Your Soul—One Day at a Time! 🌿

A clock had been running for a long, long time on the mantel piece. One day the clock began to think about how many times it would have to tick during the coming year. It counted up the seconds: 31,536,000 in one year! The old clock just got too tired and said, "I can't do it." It stopped right then and there.

When somebody reminded the clock that it didn't have to tick the 31,536,000 seconds all at once but rather one by one, the clock began to run again, and everything was all right.

One day at a time, dear caregiver!

Many times every day, go to the spa for your soul. Bring your prayers before your heavenly Father and be *still* . . . *listen* . . . *linger* . . . and then enter your day JOY-filled!

> *Dear Caregiver,* One thing that I learned as a frazzled caregiver was to purposely **S.T.O.P.** or **S**tart **T**aking **O**ccasional **P**auses. I needed time out to be *still* with the Lord. After all, my car won't run on empty and neither can I. Being *still* even for a few minutes to pray or read a verse of Scripture connected me to the ultimate power Source, Jesus Christ, and calmed my frazzled nerves.
>
> *Annetta*

Eating Concerns

Dear God,

I don't know why I'm so tired.

Dad called. He can't remember how to boil water in the
microwave.

> After I gave him very simple and specific details, he
> thought he'd try again.
> Dad called a second time. "Can you come over? I can't
> heat my coffee!"
> Before I left, I needed energy, so I gulped down a slice
> of lemon meringue pie.

He'd also asked me to pick up some apples at the grocery
store.

> I hopped in the car, and it wouldn't start.
> Oh, please, Lord, *help*!
> Meanwhile, I ate two small candy bars to calm my
> nerves.

Sure enough, Dad had his coffee hot by the time I arrived.
    "Where've you been?" he asked.
    While I sorted out his pills, I nibbled on donuts.
    He's a diabetic. He shouldn't be eating them anyway!

"What's for dinner?" he asked. *Dinner?* I'd forgotten all
  about that.
    As I rushed home, I called the kids to ask what they
      wanted
    on their hamburgers and fries.

I'm tired! I'm tired of being "on call" day and night!
    Am I the only tired caregiver?

I'm listening . . .

> ***I love You,***
> ***Your Drained Child***

. . . And God is faithful; he will not let you be tempted beyond
what you can bear. But when you are tempted,
he will also provide a way out . . .
—1 Corinthians 10:13

Eating Concerns

My Child,

You are not alone, my precious one. Caregiving is stressful,
and *you do get tired!*
  Even though each caregiver's circumstances are differ-
    ent, and many factors
  affect their energy levels, one of the common problems
    comes from food.

Caregivers have control over very little, so eating becomes a
way of doing something
  for themselves. Comfort foods and those sweets high
    in carbohydrates
  give quick energy, but they don't last.
  Come to Me for your comfort.

Becoming *aware* of some nutritional changes will help your
energy level.
  Good eating habits include eating protein and having
    sustained energy.

This is not about weight loss or gain. You need to be a
healthy caregiver!
  If you think you have no time to take care of yourself
    now,
  sooner or later you will have to find time for illness.
  If you can't take care of your loved one or yourself,
    who will?

Making changes is like having surgery. It's painful after the
operation, but then it gets better.
  Change comes by not making excuses.

An invalid had lain by the pool for thirty-eight years. Jesus
asked him if he wanted to get well.
  The invalid said, "I have no one to help me . . .
    someone else goes down ahead of me."

Jesus said, "Get up! Pick up your mat and walk." At once, the man was cured.

Believe that change can happen!

My dear, you have a beautiful servant heart! Remember, your energy level comes from what you eat.

I love you,
God

Then Jesus declared, "I am the bread of life. He who comes to me will never go hungry, and he who believes in me will never be thirsty."
—John 6:35

Today, walk in the JOY of God's Word!

Read about the invalid man in John 5:1–10.

I am sending him to you for the express purpose that you may know about our circumstances and that he may encourage your hearts.
—Colossians 4:8

Do not be anxious about anything, but in everything, by prayer and petition, with thanksgiving, present your requests to God.
—Philippians 4:6

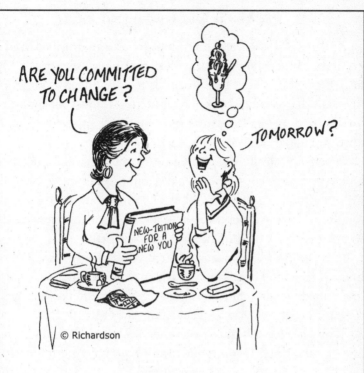

The Turn Around

I am not an addict,
 my habit I can break.
A little sundae now and then,
 what difference does it make?
I will get committed,
 and shape a brand-new me,
by ordering a single scoop,
 instead of having three.

—George Richardson

Biblical Inspiration: 1 Corinthians 10:23

✨ Who Is Your Encourager? ✨

At three o'clock every afternoon my energy dropped, and I needed a nap. I followed that with sweets to give me energy! My heart was saying, "Eat healthy foods for prolonged energy." In my head the voice said, "It doesn't matter. It's just for today."

I've tried and failed to eat right so many times. And poor nutrition equals low energy. Can you relate?

When my family became aware of my "on call" life, they intervened as encouragers. What a blessing! They would call me daily to check on what I'd eaten. Some days they gave me tough love, while other days they were all cheers. That's exactly what I needed! Everyone needs encouragement!

In Scripture a man named Barnabas was known as "Son of Encouragement." His actions were crucial to St. Paul and Mark when they started the early churches. Encouragement from Barnabas kept these men going when either could have failed (Acts 9–15).

Who will you ask to be your cheerleaders to encourage you one day at a time? Begin today through prayer. And remember that healthy caregivers commit, communicate, and connect for renewed energy:

Commit to take care of your body, God's dwelling place.

- God has a *plan* for you and a *purpose* for your life. It doesn't matter if you know what it is, He does! If He didn't have everything good planned for you, why did His Son, Jesus Christ, die in *your* place?

- Commit to eating a balanced diet and to exercising. Both provide energy!

- Commit to take action *today*!

Communicate through prayer.

- Pray for strength and perseverance to resist Satan's temptations.

- Pray for a family member, friend, or counselor you can *trust* and with whom you can *confidently* share your concerns. Getting to the emotional root of your stress and eating concerns will enable you to make positive changes.
- Pray each time before you eat and snack. Yes, before each snack!
- Pray for forgiveness when you fail. Learn to forgive yourself. Perfection is only in heaven!
- Praise God for your successes and your encouragers.

Connect with your encouragers.

- Talk to your encourager often. Ask for tough love to hold you accountable when you've made poor choices.
- Talk and listen to God for guidance and strength. Read His Word daily.[7]
- The JOY of God's presence will be your strength!

Dear Caregiver, Here's a list of energizing grab-and-go snacks that we keep in the house and car: almonds, walnuts, protein bars, string cheese, fresh fruit, carrots, and other fresh veggies. If you have nut allergies, beef sticks are a great alternative. Drink lots of water, beginning with God's Living Water! Take a walk, even if it's just in the house. If you need an encourager, have food tips to share, or if you want to receive *Nuggets of Hope* newsletters, contact us at joy4caringhearts@gmail.com.

Annetta and Karen

Just as God enables you to rise to each new challenge, trust that He will equip you, [dear caregiver], with the resources you need at the appropriate time.

—Author Unknown

Equipped for a Purpose

Dear God,

As I sit here rocking my three-year-old, I am so grateful
   that he is alive
      and now home from the hospital.
      At the same time, I feel like I'm walking in a fog.
      Where does the journey go from here?

My husband and I were elated that after two girls You gave
   us a boy.
      We could see ourselves watching him play T-ball and
         later
      cheering for him as quarterback of his high school
         football team.

Now it seems our life is one question after another.
      Are there other parents who have had a child suffer a
         stroke?
      How will we manage a feeding tube? What if it gets
         clogged?
      Will he get enough nourishment?
      Will we have to change diapers forever?

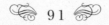

It may seem selfish, but as a couple we have questions, too:
    Will we be able to afford the continuous medical
        expenses?
    Will the girls feel neglected?
    Will we ever experience living as empty-nesters?

Lord, I'm scared.
    I'm so overwhelmed and feel inadequate to be in a
        caregiving role!
    Where do I start?

I am listening . . .

I love You,
Your Inadequate Child

When I said, "My foot is slipping," your love, O LORD,
supported me. When anxiety was great within me,
your consolation brought joy to my soul.
—Psalm 94:18–19

Equipped for a Purpose

My Child,

Come into my open arms as I embrace your broken heart.

- *Feel* My powerful strength sustaining you night and day!
- *Hear* My almighty voice, which has, is, and always will continue to guide you.
- *Believe* in My promises. I am faithful to *every single one.*
- *Trust* in Me. I will never allow you to walk this journey alone.

Remember your favorite Bible story when you were a little girl? You asked your mother to read
it to you over and over again. It was about a man who was robbed, beaten, and left on the
roadside while on his way to Jericho. Do you think he could have felt hopeless because
neither the priest nor Levite stopped to help him? It was the Samaritan, the one least expected to help, who put *love into action.*

One of the ways I will equip you is through "good Samaritans," who will personally put My
love into *action* as your faith is tested. They'll give you comfort and encouragement to persevere. These "good Samaritans" are my *God-surprises* in your day!

When you least expect it, "good Samaritans" will become specialists, caring teachers, and
physical therapists providing resources you never could have found on your own.
You'll be amazed at how friends will say encouraging words at exactly the right moment.
Your church family will intercede through prayer.
Their hugs will be My hugs.

And don't be surprised when some "good Samaritan"
  leaves a pizza by your front door
on the *exact* day you are mentally and physically
  burned out.

Precious caregiver, I know you are suddenly looking at life
  from a new perspective.
    The boundaries of your world have shifted from what
      was so secure to uncertainties.
    Trust in Me rather than dwelling on why.

Never forget that I am *your* caregiver. My presence will be
  the *real* JOY in your journey.
    With all that I have done for your *eternal* relationship
      with Me,
    do you really think I'd allow anything in this temporal
      world that could truly defeat you?

I love you,
God

Consider it pure joy, my brothers, whenever you face trials of
many kinds, because you know that the testing of your faith
develops perseverance.
—James 1:2–3

Today, walk in the JOY of God's Word!

Read the Good Samaritan story in Luke 10:30–37.

May the God of peace, equip you with everything good for
doing his will, and may he work in us what is pleasing to him,
through Jesus Christ . . .
—Hebrew 13:20

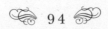

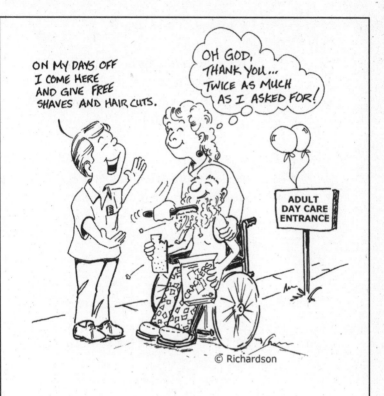

Surprise

God is good all the time.
        He wants the same from me.
And as I give my care to them,
        His workings I will see.
Pouring out to overflow,
        the blessing as it rises,
and when the need is truly great,
        He gives His best surprises.
                                —*George Richardson*

Biblical Inspiration: Luke 6:38

❧ "Someone Who Cares"[8] ❧

So often I've thought of me
Putting myself first so selfishly
Looking through eyes that only saw my point of view
And not you.

Then someone reached out to me
When I needed compassion desperately
I saw the truth and suddenly knew that
You need me to be
Someone who cares.

I want to have Your heart
When somebody else's breaks apart
Ready to serve
Letting Your Word lead the way
Every day
Someone who cares.

Someone who's willing to stand tall
when the rain falls
Someone who cares
Someone who's there for the long haul
An answer to just one prayer
Help me to be
Someone who cares.

—Words and Music
by Scott Krippayne and Steve Siler

Equipped for a Purpose

Dear Caregiver, We keep this thought, written on a card, taped on our refrigerators and in our cars to remind us not to worry. We encourage you to do this, too.

Four simple ways to handle worry:

Presence: Claim God's presence. Say to yourself, "I'm not alone."

Promises: Recount God's promises. There are over 7,000 of them in the Scriptures.

Prayer: Tell God about your worry. After doing so, leave it with Him!

Patience: Wait on God. Rather than rushing in, trust in His provision.

Source Unknown

Annetta and Karen

Lay your burdens at the foot of the cross, [dear caregiver], and ask God to open minds and soften hearts as He impresses upon everyone His wishes and will.

—Charles Puchta

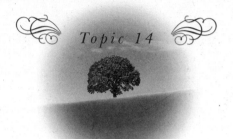

Family Conflict

Dear God,

I am *angry*!
>   I don't want to think about all of this,
>   much less have to help anyone solve anything!

Lately the twins have been arguing all the time.
>   I know they're teenagers, but it's wearing on my nerves.
>   Yesterday they argued about whose turn it was to drive
>   to school.
>   I made them ride the bus instead. They haven't talked
>   to me yet.

My oldest announced that he's losing his job.
>   Now he's moving back home.

My youngest needs a costume for the school play.
>   When am I going to have the time to come up with that?
>   She seems to think I'm mean because I'm not jumping
>   up and down
>   over her good fortune in having been chosen.
>   I feel like the meanest mom in town!

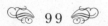

I'm just tired of dealing with conflict, Lord.
> I don't think I can handle many more problems.

I'm drained of energy, having to juggle all the family
  conflict
> *plus* take care of my father who lives in the next state!
> My sister and I disagree on how to take care of him.
> That's a whole issue by itself!

I need your help, Lord!

I'm listening . . .

> ### *I love You,*
> ### *Your Child of Unrest*

*Answer me when I call to you, O my righteous God. Give me
relief from my distress; be merciful to me and hear my prayer.*
—Psalm 4:1

Family Conflict

My Child,

Why are you so angry?
> Family conflicts have always been and will continue to
> be in the world.
> Why? Because of *sin*!

Cain and Abel had family conflict.
> The result? The first murder.

Isaac favored Esau; Rebekah favored Jacob.
> The result? Trickery, deceit, and friction.

Leah and Rachel were tokens used by their father to finish
deals.
> The result? Jealousy and ridicule.

Many examples exist in the Scriptures.
> And even when they ended in defeat or disappointments,
> My faithfulness never wavered for those who loved Me.

My faithfulness will never waiver for you either.
> Be assured that you can place your confidence in Me
> because I will listen when you call.
> I listen to your prayers, and
> I will always answer them
> in My time.

David called upon me and was
impatient, thinking I hadn't
answered him in a timely
manner.
> However, he trusted Me and
> showed steadfast faith in
> My unfailing love.

Family conflicts often
revolve around issues
of power.

Sometimes all you may need is to talk over a problem with
a trusted friend, pastor,
or counselor to help put it into perspective.
Family conflicts often revolve around issues of power.

One thing to keep in mind is that the JOY of my presence
will always be your strength for any conflict you face.
I am always here for you!

I love you,
God

But I trust in your unfailing love; my heart rejoices in your
salvation. I will sing to the Lord, for he has been good to me.
—Psalm 13:5–6

Today, walk in the JOY of God's Word!

Read about Cain's story in Genesis 4:1–17.
Read about Isaac and Rebekah and the blessing in Genesis 27.
Read about Leah and Rachel in Genesis 29:15–30.

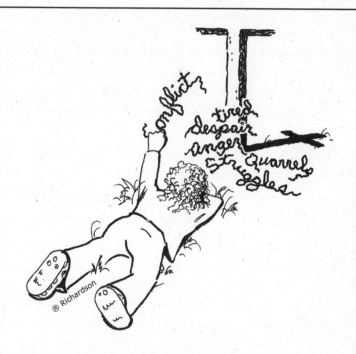

My Yoke

I was an ox,
    who pulled a plow,
        of anger and despair.
At the cross,
    I put it down,
        and left my conflict there.
Thanks to Him,
    who knew my need,
        and revealed it to my sight.
I now possess,
    a yoke of ease,
        My burden now is light.

                    —*George Richardson*

Biblical Inspiration: Matthew 11:28–30

❧ Conflict Resolution Tips ❧

C **Communicate** effectively. Talk so that the other person will be able to listen to your *heart*. Don't start the conversation in a harsh and accusing way so as to make the other person defensive. Take time to cool down from strong emotional reactions.

O **Openly** resolve conflict in a healthy, respectful way. Don't sacrifice the relationship over a situation.

N **Never** try to change family members—recognize their strengths and weaknesses and accept them for who they are.

F **Feelings** of resentment can escalate if you don't deal with them. Overextending yourself can make you tired and cause bitterness and an unwillingness to forgive. Recognize your feelings, and then constructively communicate how you feel and *what you need*.

L **Live your prayer life**. Be honest with God about how you feel, releasing your initial strong emotions. Then ask God to fill you with His Spirit and enable you to have a loving and helpful attitude in your heart.

I **Intervention** by a professional (mediator) may be needed if you aren't able to resolve conflicts. The mediator could be a family member you trust, a good friend, or a pastor. A counselor also might be helpful.

C **Connect** regularly with family members about a parent's condition via routine e-mail messages, letters, texts, or phone calls.

T **Take time out** to calm down and get to the bottom of what you are *really* feeling. Do not just vent your anger and say harsh, wounding, and unproductive words. Take a walk.

Breathe deeply. Journal. Go for counseling. After you feel the initial intensity of your emotions has calmed down, then you can go back and talk and resolve the issue with the other person.[9]

Dear Caregiver, When we were caregivers, it was so easy to fall into the trap of anger, frustration, and unresolved feelings with a loved one, a family member, or someone else. These tips helped us, and we hope they're useful in your caregiving life.

Annetta and Karen

There's no "perfect" way to give care, [dear care-giver]. Perfection isn't the goal. Love is!

—Author Unknown

Failure

Dear God,

I blew it, and I knew it!
> I wrote the check for the oxygen tank out of the wrong
> account, *again*.
> Hopefully, the car insurance isn't due until next
> month.

I can't remember tomorrow's doctor's appointment time.
> I wrote it down, but I can't find my note.
> Will they recognize my voice if I call *again*?

I used *that voice tone* when the tomato juice was spilled,
again.
> The carpet is already thread-bare.

I can't do anything right!
> I'm not helping my loved one, only frustrating him.
> I'm not helping my family; I'm not there for them.
> Most of all, God, I'm not helping *me*.

My heart is breaking into shards of glass that are
    piercing my soul with guilt, fear, and frustration.
      What am I to do? I only know that I'm on my knees
        before you, Lord,
      because You are the only one I can talk to about this.

If only I could keep one step ahead of things, but I only
  manage
      to fall further behind.

I just want to give up. *I'm a failure*!

Is there any hope for me?

I'm listening . . .

                I love You,
                Your Failing-at-Life Child

My heart throbs; my strength fails me,
and the light of my eyes—it also has gone from me.
—Psalm 38:10

My Child,

Oh, my precious child, come into My arms and let Me
reassure you.
I see all that you are doing for your loved one.
You are making a difference in his life!

Let all your concerns about your failures be forgotten
in the real JOY of My mercy and faithfulness.

Refresh your soul as you read from the Scriptures about
others who felt that they, too, had failed.
How do you think Moses felt when he came down
from the mountain with the stone tablets of Law
in his arms, only to see that the very people he was
leading had gone back to their worship of a golden
calf?

What about Peter, the rock on whom I would build My
church?
There were times when he felt that he had failed My
Son, especially when, out of fear for his own safety,
he denied even knowing
Jesus after the temple
guards had arrested Him.

Walk in their footsteps. See the
humanity of My followers.
You can see their mistakes,
yet you can rejoice in
seeing My forgiveness, too.

You can rejoice
in seeing My
forgiveness.

Drink daily from My well of
Living Water, where you will be refreshed
from lessons full of encouragement and hope that
reflect the JOY of my presence.

My faithfulness is a promise to you!
My promises to the faithful shine brightly by bringing
hope
for tomorrow and strength for today.

I love you!
God

*For everything that was written in the past was written to
teach us, so that through endurance and the encouragement of
Scriptures we might have hope.*
—Romans 15:4

Today, walk in the JOY of God's Word!

Read about Moses in Exodus 32.
Read about Peter's denial of Jesus in Matthew 26:69–75
and John 21:15–22.

*But I will sing of your strength; I will sing aloud of your
steadfast love in the morning. For you have been to me a
fortress and a refuge in the day of my distress.*
—Psalm 59:16

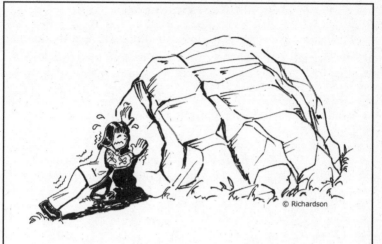

© Richardson

Faithful

Am I just a loser,
      pushing on this rock?
Maybe I am stronger,
      but moving it is not.
Thank God He doesn't measure,
      successes never meant.
Only that we're faithful,
      to Jesus whom He sent.
                    —*George Richardson*

Biblical Inspiration: Psalm 31:23

❧ Keep Pushing ❧

Has Satan ever used his tool of making you feel inadequate to discourage you? To be human is to feel inadequate! Our Enemy uses every creative tool in his bag to make us think we can do everything ourselves and that if we can't, we are failures. A modern-day parable explains it this way:

> Once upon a time the Lord appeared to a woman. He explained that He had work for her to do. Daily she was to push with all her strength against the massive rock in her yard.
>
> She served the Lord joyfully, doing the task daily, until Satan started playing mind games with her. "Didn't the Lord say you should move the rock? You are inadequate for the job. You are a failure!" taunted the Enemy.
>
> She was ready to give up because she was burned-out from the same daily routine, but first she decided to make it a matter of prayer.
>
> God said to her, "My child, you have done just as I asked. You may not have thought anything was happening, but you can always trust the plans I have for you. You have listened and done what I asked you to do—push the rock. You are now stronger. I have been strengthening you to meet the challenges in your daily walk."

Jesus, the Rock of your salvation, asks you to press forward in your journey, totally trusting Him. Remember, feeling inadequate or helpless doesn't mean hopelessness. With man, there is a hopeless end; but with God, there will always be endless hope!

Failure

There are many stories of people in the Bible who struggled with feeling inadequate. Remember the story of Queen Esther? She may have felt inadequate approaching the king without permission. But had God strengthened her for such a time as that? Yes! (See Esther 4.)

Let your faith guide you to look at what Christ has done in the past when you feel inadequate. Apply that faith to your caregiving. Make the blessings of the past an injection of JOY to revitalize your discouraged heart. Keep pushing!

Dear Caregiver, No one can do it all. Perfection is only in heaven! Just do the best you can and leave the rest to God.

Annetta and Karen

Nobody knows what is around the corner of tomorrow but you can be certain, [dear caregiver], that God will be waiting there for you. Never give up hope! God's mercies are new each morning.

—Jill Brisco

Financial Crisis

Dear God,

Each day becomes more of a challenge with our finances!
Help me to stay focused on the fact that You will give
me wisdom on what to do.
Satan is working overtime to make me discouraged.

I shoulder all the responsibilities of overseeing my husband's care,
our household, and paying the bills.

I'm praying I won't lose my job.
We need those health benefits. Prescription costs keep
rising.
How can we afford to keep paying such high costs?

Our car is ten years old, and the repairs are endless.
Can a fuel pump really cost that much?

The rent is due.
We can't be using that much electricity, can we?

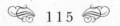

My retirement portfolio has been cut in half.
 I've about used up all our savings.
  Would I have enough energy to work a second job?

It broke my heart today, God, when he smiled and said,
 "Honey, I appreciate all you do. Somehow we'll make
 it. If only I could help."

What can I do?

I'm listening . . .

    I love You,
    Your Very Concerned Child

Trust in Him at all times, O people; pour out your hearts to
Him; for God is our refuge.
  —Psalm 62:8

Financial Crisis

My Child,

I'm so glad you have come to Me with your concerns.
    I love you and want only good for you.
    Fix your eyes on Me, dear child, and you will
    find *endurance* for today and *hope* for tomorrow.

You have seen my faithfulness through past generations,
    and you can trust that I will keep my promises forever.
    I will provide for you in
        unexpected ways,
    just as I did for a widow
        and her two sons.

She had no idea how she
    could pay her creditors, and
    if she didn't,
        they would take her sons
        to be slaves as payment.
    All she had was one jar of
        olive oil! So she went
        to Elisha for help.

Fix your eyes on Me,
dear child, and you will
find *endurance* for today
and hope for tomorrow.

Elisha told her to go and ask all her neighbors for a lot of
    empty jars.
    She filled all the containers from her one jar of oil
        before it stopped flowing.
    Elisha told her to sell all the jars of oil, pay her debts,
        and live on the rest of the money.

She asked Elisha for help because she recognized his
    devotion to Me.
    Her faith never wavered. She knew and loved Me.

Trust every detail of your life to Me, and take advantage of
    the many resources I provide for you.
    I have promised to meet all your needs according to
        My glorious riches.

Find JOY in My presence, even during difficult and
  costly times.
Have faith, My child. I am with you *always*.

I love you,
God

The steadfast love of the LORD never ceases;
his mercies never come to an end;
they are new every morning; great is your faithfulness.
—Lamentations 3:22–23 ESV

Today, walk in the JOY of God's Word!

Read about the widow and Elisha in 2 Kings 4:1–7.

And he said to the woman,
"Your faith has saved you; go in peace."
—Luke 7:50 ESV

God is our refuge and strength, an ever-present help in trouble.
—Psalms 46:1

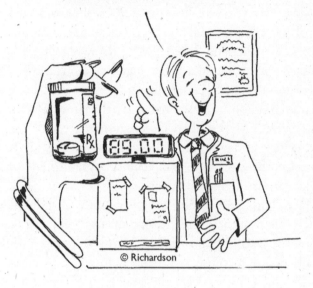

In Him I Trust

The cost is steep,
   it seems unfair,
      even with the Medicare.
But God owns all upon the hills,
   which is enough to pay the bills.
     In Him my trust I'll keep.
         —*George Richardson*

Biblical Inspiration: Psalm 32:10 and Psalm 50:10

❧ Who Can Help? ❧

Joann couldn't wait to share her new recipe for sugar-free cookies with her good friend and neighbor, Mary. Joann walked in the back door as usual but gasped as she took in the scene before her. There was her friend, lying on the floor.

"Mary! Mary!" she called out as she rushed and knelt at the side of her friend. "Mary, can you hear me?" Joann made a quick assessment and called 9-1-1. Knowing that Mary was a diabetic, she wondered if her sugar count was low. Was she going into a diabetic coma? Joann found a little bit of sugar and put some on Mary's tongue. By the time the emergency squad arrived, Mary still lay unconscious.

After several days in the hospital, Mary was ready to be released. On the way home Joann timidly asked, "Did you forget to take your medicine that day?"

Mary's body wilted. She sheepishly said, "I didn't have the money this month to order a prescription refill, so I've been cutting the pills in half to make them last longer. I didn't tell the ER doctor because I was too embarrassed. Sometimes I wonder where my retirement money goes. Everything is so expensive these days!"

Joann pulled into a mall parking lot, stopped the car, and turned to her friend. "Mary, I am your friend. If you're having difficulty with anything, confide in me. I want to help you, but if you don't share these things with me, I won't know that you need help. I know some places to contact, so let's go home and make a plan. I know there are resources available, and we will take the time to look into this *together*. Let's pray right now to have God guide us in our searching."

If God can use a boy with a small stone to kill a Philistine giant, then you know how much He can help you in any difficulty you're having. Just as His love and faithfulness were with

David when he killed Goliath, His love and faithfulness are with you in all that you do. That's real JOY, and it's there in spite of circumstances.

Dear Caregiver, God surrounds us with people who can help, but we have to reach out to them. Here are some ideas that may help:

- Use a small notebook. Journal the date, telephone number, and information that you find helpful. Write down every lead and follow up on them. Keep your journal up-to-date because you may need the information again.

- Tell your family doctor that the high cost of your prescriptions is too much for you. He could look into another, less-expensive prescription; a generic brand; or give you some free samples.

- Helpful resources: contact your pastor, local senior service agency, financial planners. Social workers from the hospital can help you find financial aid to help with your medical expenses.

- Local resources: food bank, utility companies for smaller monthly payments, a neighbor who could give you a discount on your car repairs.[10]

Annetta and Karen

On the cross, Jesus prayed, "Father forgive them," even though no one said, "I'm sorry."

—Author Unknown

Forgiveness

Dear God,

How can I do this one more day?
    I'm ready to walk out of here and never come back!

Let me tell You about today.
    Dirty adult diapers were changed non-stop.
    She refuses to take her medicine. It went flying across
        the room.
    The food she didn't like was rubbed through her hair,
        smeared on her face,
    and then thrown on the floor.

This week she was back teaching school and was even using
    the students' names.
        This lasted for three days *and* nights, and then she was
            exhausted and
        slept continuously. (Forgive me, Lord, for rejoicing
            about those hours
        of peace and quiet!)

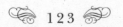

My brothers and sisters-in-law keep an eye on me like a
hawk.
>They want to make sure I do everything just right, and
>>yet they refuse to help.
>(I admit, and You already know, that I'm sometimes
>>"too busy" when I see whose
>name is on my caller I.D. . . . I'm too exhausted to be
>>interrogated again.)

Honestly, Lord, I have all these emotions flying around
inside of me,
>especially because of how she abused me as a child.
>And yet, deep down my spirit wants to forgive her.
>I want to be free from this anguish.

Help me!

I'm listening . . .

>>>*I love You,*
>>>***Your Heavy-hearted Child***

*Bear with each other and forgive whatever grievances you may
have against one another. Forgive as the Lord forgave you.*
>—Colossians 3:13

My Child,

Of course, your natural response is to throw stones at those
who hurt you rather than to forgive.
Yet, I know *your* heart and how this heavy burden
continually
wears you down, both mentally and physically.

Forgiveness is not
forgetting, being weak, or excusing the wrong.
It is taking the grievance
off *your* hook and
totally placing it on
Me.

Forgiveness is
grace that flows *to* you
from Me and *through*
you *to* others,
and understanding the
depth of my *uncondi-
tional* love for you, dear
caregiver.

When you decide to
forgive someone, it is an
action that will result
in a *freedom* like you've
never felt before!

When you decide to forgive someone, it is an action that
will result in a
freedom like you've never felt before!
To hear the words of forgiveness is to hear JOY and
gladness.
How liberating!

When you pray, "Forgive us our debts, as we also have
forgiven our debtors" (Matt. 6:12),
you are asking Me to forgive you in the exact same way
that
you have forgiven those who have wronged you.

I will never keep a list of your offenses. What do you
    do with *your* lists?
Do you keep your lists or dump your bag of burdens at
    the foot of the cross?

Your choice does *not* have to depend on the offender's
    readiness to respond,
        but *solely* on *your* willingness to release your
        resentment.
        As you release these unwanted thoughts, replace them
        with My grace-filled Word!

There is great JOY in *being* forgiven and *in* forgiving others.

I love you,
God

Let us then approach the throne of grace with confidence,
so that we may receive mercy and find grace to help us
in our time of need.
—Hebrews 4:16

Today, walk in the JOY of God's Word!

[Jesus said], "For God so loved the world that he gave his one
and only Son, that whoever believes in him shall not perish
but have eternal life. For God did not send his Son
into the world to condemn the world, but
to save the world through him."
—John 3:16–17

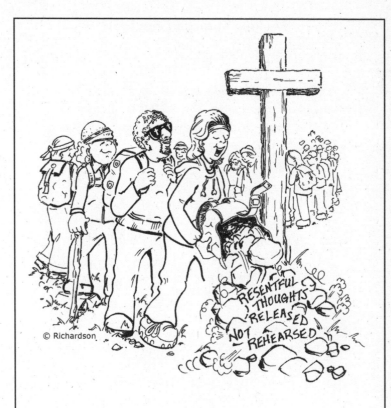

Tossed Out

Not all sins hang from our back,
    there for all to see.
Jesus said within our thoughts,
    the equal danger be.
Like a sack we open up,
    confess, repent, release.
Tossing out unrighteousness,
    and then we walk in peace.

—*George Richardson*

Biblical Inspiration: 1 John 1:5–10

🍃 Looking Through *Cross* Eyes 🍃

Think about this hypothetical story:

> A van pulls up in front of your home. The driver knocks on your door and says, "This is a free DVD just for you!" With curiosity, you read the title, "This Is Your Life," and play it immediately.

The DVD contains every detail about you:

... your first breath, first tooth, first step, first kiss.

... your broken toe and all those paper cuts on your left thumb.

... the fun as well as the sad times with family and friends.

... the kind as well as the hurtful words you've said.

... every thought you've had, including those you would never want anyone to know.

> Jesus already knows *every* detail about your life, and He ... *still* ... *loves ... you*!

> There's not one thing missing from the movie of your life. There are even details about today, when you confessed your sins and asked for forgiveness for when you ...

If this happened, how many people would you want to show *your* "life movie" to?

Jesus already knows *every* detail about your life, and He ... *still* ... *loves* ... *you*! Seeing yourself from the cross, as Jesus sees you, is looking through the eyes of grace!

Would looking through *cross* eyes radically change the way you think of God's grace?

Forgiveness

Go to God and
Rest in His faithfulness,
Assured of His everlasting love and
Comforted with His promise of
Eternal life.

Dear Caregiver, Knowing that God has forgiven you is outrageous, ecstatic, everlasting JOY! Here are the steps we use as a guide to help us forgive:

- Acknowledge and give your thoughts to God (Ps. 147:3).

- Meditate on God's Word, because it heals the hurts in your heart (Ps. 107:20).

- Use the power tool of praise to replace your negative thoughts (Ps. 43:5).

- Pray. It redirects your heart (Col. 3:13).

- Focus on this fact: God's forgiveness has nothing to do with the offense, but everything to do with Him (1 Cor. 13:5).

Annetta and Karen

Have you noticed, [dear caregiver], how God will bring a person or a circumstance into your life to encourage you at the very moment you're ready to give in to despair?

—Dale Crawshaw

Friends

Dear God,

Shockwaves have plummeted to the depths of my soul.
My close friend just called with her test results.

I thought I was prepared to hear this kind of news, but I'm
not.
The tears won't stop.
I feel so helpless, and yet I have such inner peace.
I know You will be holding her hand securely in this
new journey.

I suddenly realize that not only are her family members
caregivers,
but also, as a friend, I'm a caregiver, too.

Give me wisdom to know what to do for her.
Guide my hands to be Your hands.

Enable me, through your Holy Spirit, to speak words
of encouragement, comfort, and hope.

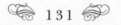

Help me share this divine truth . . .
    that the real JOY we have in our journey is Your
      constant presence.
    That will be my reservoir of strength.

Show me how to be a real friend to her.

I'm listening . . .

                     I love You,
                     Your Tear-streaked Child

A friend loves at all times.
—Proverbs 17:17

Friends

My Child,

Friends are most definitely caregivers, too!

It is no accident that the two
   of you have been friends for
   many years.
      I have watched you cry
         together, rejoice together,
         and
      even laugh until your sides
         hurt with silliness.

Friends are most
definitely caregivers,
too!

Do not doubt that I will work as
   a caregiver in your friendship.
      I created you. You are uniquely you!
      Your gifts and talents will minister to her in ways that
         only I know.
      Be an open vessel, and follow the nudges of the Holy Spirit.

You are the salt of the earth.
      You bring a different flavor to her life and will be a
         difference-maker in this
         journey.
      You will be My hands, so
         reach out and touch them
         with My love.

You will be My
hands, so reach out
and touch them with
My love.

Draw strength for this journey
   by remembering David and
   Jonathan's friendship.
      Jonathan saved David's life.
      And at their final parting,
         they kissed and wept together.
      I was a witness of their friendship.

A friend is not afraid to feel the pain of others.
  Be a witness of the depth of My love.
  My Son gave His life for those whom He loved.

As you share the Good News and JOY of your salvation
  together,
    continue to laugh, cry, rejoice,
    and listen . . . especially listen.

I love you,
God

. . . for the joy of the LORD is your strength.
—Nehemiah 8:10b

Today, walk in the JOY of God's Word!

Peace to you. The friends here send their greetings.
Greet the friends there by name.
—3 John 1:15

[Jesus said], "For where two or three come together
in my name, there am I with them."
—Matthew 18:20

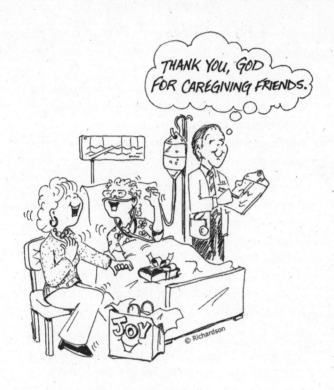

Friends

We have so much in common,
     collected through the years,
sharing all the good times,
     and comfort in our fears.
You and me with Jesus,
     He showed us how to live,
through sacrificial living,
     by friends who care to give.
          —George Richardson

Biblical Inspiration: John 15:12–17

🐚 Where's My Help? 🐚

Have you ever thought about who would carry your cot if you needed help? Read this story, written by Rev. Bob Willis:

Jesus was in Capernaum teaching the people. He was in a house with a crowd of people standing all around him. They even overflowed out the doorway! Everyone wanted to hear and see Jesus as He taught the Word to those who listened.

The Bible records there were four men carrying a paralyzed friend on a bed. They wanted to put their friend in front of Jesus so that He would heal him. But when they arrived at the home they couldn't get in because of all the people. So they climbed onto the roof of the house, took some roof tiles off, and lowered their friend down through the ceiling to the feet of Jesus.

When Jesus saw their faith, He forgave the sins of their friend. The scribes were thinking in their heart that Jesus was committing blasphemy by forgiving sins. They had not said a word, but Jesus read their hearts. He proved His power by not only forgiving the man's sins, but also healing his sick body. Jesus said, "I tell you, get up, take your mat and go home." Immediately he rose and walked away.

This amazed everyone and they praised God, saying, "We have never seen anything like this!" Perhaps they were amazed at the large crowd, maybe they were amazed at the teaching of Jesus or the way the four men took time to bring their friend to Jesus, or the manner in which they removed the roof tiles and lowered their friend through the ceiling. Or perhaps they were amazed that Jesus forgave his sins, or that Jesus healed the paralyzed man. Regardless of their point of amazement, it was definitely God at work in their midst![11]

What if *you* were the one on the bed, the one so sick you had to depend on others to carry you? Name someone who could hold one corner of your bed. It would take at least four people to carry you on the bed, one on each corner. Do you have at least four people you could rely on to be there for you? Count it all JOY that you can name *your* caregivers.

As a caregiver, do not be afraid to ask for help.

As a caregiver, do not be afraid to ask for help. After all, these friends knew they needed each other in order to take their friend to Jesus. If even one had failed in the task, it would have made it more difficult, if not impossible, for the others. God honors teamwork, and He honors you as a caregiver. Never be afraid to ask for help.

Dear Caregiver, Now imagine your loved one on the bed, and you are holding one corner. Your loved one is depending on you to support and carry him/her while not being able to care for himself/herself. Can you list three others to help you carry the load? The load is too heavy for one caregiver; you need help, and you need others.

Annetta and Karen

Laughter does not mean you are ignoring pain, living in denial, or just not aware of the troubles around you. For me, laughter is how we take a much-needed break from the heartache, so that when we turn to face it again, it has by some miracle grown smaller in size and intensity, if not disappeared altogether.

—Liz Curtis Higgs

Topic 19

Humor

Dear God,

Were You laughing last Sunday when I said,
   "Give ear to my prayer, O Lord, consider my
      medication?"
   Sorry, I really meant to say *meditation.*[12]

Someone at church must know how stressed I am from
   going to the
      nursing home every afternoon because a package was
         left in my car.
      The note on the *JOY Box* said, "Take this with you to
         the nursing home.
      Remove one or two items each day.
      Enjoy reading them to your wife and others, and see
         what happens!"
      A Good Samaritan[13]

Oh, thank You, Lord, for whoever thought of doing this
   for us.
      The laughter, giggles, little snickers, and even those
         quiet inner vibes

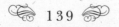

that spread through our mind and body helped to
lighten our spirits.
This was great medicine! We decided there isn't
much fun in medicine,
but there's a lot of medicine in fun.

Thank You, Lord, for creating the gift of laughter!
It relaxes us. When my wife is relaxed, then *I* relax.

My problem is that I'm feeling guilty for enjoying this
light-heartedness.
Is this okay? Do You like humor?

I'm listening . . .

> *I love You,*
> *Your Relaxed Child*

A joyful heart is good medicine,
but a crushed spirit dries up the bones.
—Proverbs 17:22 ESV

Humor

My Child,

I love talking to you, dearest one, and hearing your
   thoughts and questions.
   I love to smile when I look at you!

Don't feel guilty. Humor is a way to release tension and
   help people cope.
   When humor is *used* with warmth and sensitivity,
   it expresses our *compassion* and caring.
   Have you noticed how your loved one occasionally
      uses humor
   to convey a serious concern?

I know the *stress* you experience as a caregiver.
   Because of what stress can do to your health, those
      light-hearted times are critical.
   They help to *balance* the more serious times when your
      responsibilities weigh heavily.

King Solomon knew the value of laughter when he said,
   "There is a time for everything and a season for every
      activity under heaven . . .
   a time to weep and a time to laugh" (Eccles. 3:1,4).
   You are not laughing *at* someone's hardships, you are
      laughing to *get through* them.

Humor therapy is a valuable tool for good health.
   It produces the body's natural pain killer (endorphins)
   and strengthens the immune system.
   Circulation and digestion are improved. Blood pres-
      sure is lowered.
   The more relaxed you are, the less likely you are to be
      argumentative.[14]

You asked if I like humor. What do you think?
  My Son hid a coin in a fish's mouth.
  When Jesus turned water into wine at the wedding
    feast,
  do you think there was joy and laughter?
  Watching many of the things you do brings JOY to my
    heart!

You may not realize it, but people notice My presence
  through your JOY-filled witness.
    You reflect *hope* in My faithfulness.
    Your life of faith produces JOY because it has the *right*
      focus.

I love you,
God

I have told you this so that my joy may be in you
and that your joy may be complete.
—John 15:11

Today, walk in the JOY of God's Word!

Read about the wedding in Cana in John 2:1–12.

". . . go to the lake and throw out your line.
Take the first fish you catch; open its mouth and
you will find a four-drachma coin."
—Matthew 17:27

He will yet fill your mouth with laughter and
your lips with shouts of joy.
—Job 8:21

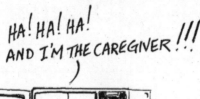

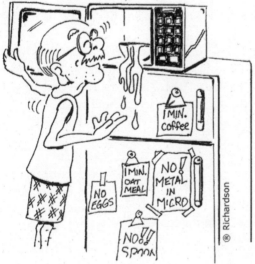

Big Thanks

Thank the Lord for humor,
     the giggle and the laugh,
it helps relieve the stresses
     and blows away the chaff.
There remains the kernel
     of truth that Jesus saves,
so lift your hands with fervor
     and not just "micro-waves."
           —*George Richardson*

Biblical Inspiration: Proverbs 17:22

JOYzette

Weather: Sunny   Temperature: Perfect   Date: Today

MODERN DISCOVERY?

We're just now discovering what the Bible has said for thousands of years. "There is a time to weep and a time to laugh." (Ecclesiastes 3:4)

"If you're not allowed to laugh in heaven, I don't want to go there." Martin Luther (1483–1546)

Don't let your worries get the best of you; remember, Moses started out as a basket case!

While preaching a sermon, the pastor said to his congregation, "If you are happy today, I wish you'd tell your face."

HUMOROUS JOBS

My first job was working in an orange juice factory, but I got canned—couldn't concentrate. After that, I tried to be a tailor, but I just wasn't suited for it—mainly because it was a so-so job.
Next I tried working in a muffler factory, but that was exhausting.
Finally, I attempted to be a deli worker, but any way I sliced it, I couldn't cut the mustard any more.
And what would you say about the jobs you've had?

The good Lord didn't create anything without a purpose, but mosquitoes come close.

Some minds are like concrete, thoroughly mixed up and permanently set.

Dear Caregiver, We personally know the heavy burdens of caregiving, but we also appreciate God's gift of humor. Isn't it amazing how God will put someone in your day who adds just the right amount of humor to help give you a better perspective? Who would this be for you? Write and tell us how humor has helped you as a caregiver: joy4caringhearts@gmail.com.

Annetta and Karen

Stay heavenward focused, [dear caregiver], and even the giant storms of life will not be strong enough to blow you away.

—Dale Crawshaw

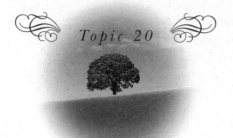

Verbal Abuse

Dear God,

I could see it coming . . .
> His breathing—rapid and deep.
> His fists—clenched.
> His lips—firmly placed in *that* position.
> His facial muscles—tight.

Here comes more verbal abuse!
> "You can *never* do anything right!"
> "Why can't you keep this house clean?"
> "Did you see the newspaper article I laid on your chair about losing weight?"
> "Get out of here, and leave me alone!"

Lord, it didn't take me long to realize how much words can hurt.
> His words are like a jagged knife wound that just won't heal.

Father, You know how hard I try to stay calm, especially
   when he gets abusive,
      but You also know how scared I am.
      Will those hurtful words turn into physical abuse?
      I just don't know what to do.

I'm listening . . .

> *I love You,*
> *Your Scared Child*

The troubles of my heart have multiplied;
   free me from my anguish.
      —Psalm 25:17

My Child,

Because you are hurting, I'm also hurting. Verbal abuse is
not what I want for you.
Let My Words comfort you, strengthen you, and bring
healing to your broken spirit.

My Words gave great comfort to David, who was in a
caregiving role himself.
David, although loved by King Saul, still experienced
challenges in giving him care.
Over time, King Saul's condition worsened, and
sometimes David feared for his life.
So much so that he asked for the help of his good
friend Jonathan.

Do not be afraid to ask for
help.
I have placed professional
people in many walks
of life who can help you
right now.
Don't be afraid to talk
with them.
There may come a time
when you will need
their help to care for
your loved one,
not only for his sake, but
also for yours.

I am faithful to My
promises to never leave
nor forsake you.
Let this assurance seep
deep into your soul and
help you find strength
for the day.

I hear you, my child. And I want you to trust Me, just as
David did.

I have loved you with an everlasting love.
Never be afraid to take refuge in the shelter of My
wings.

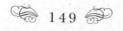

I am faithful to My promises to never leave nor forsake
you.
Let this assurance seep deep into your soul and help
you find strength for the day.
My presence will always give you JOY-filled hope.

I love you,
God

When anxiety was great within me,
your consolation brought joy to my soul.
—Psalm 94:19

Today, walk in the JOY of God's Word!

Read about David in 1 Samuel 16:14–23.

I have loved you with an everlasting love;
therefore I have continued my faithfulness to you.
—Jeremiah 31:3 ESV

Create in me a pure heart, O God,
and renew a steadfast spirit within me.
—Psalm 51:10

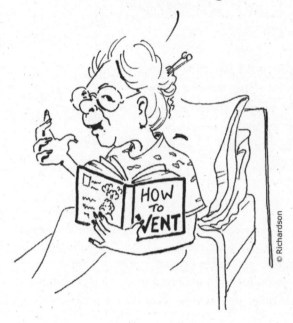

A Godly Force

By Your Spirit,
    grant me strength,
        in godly force repay.
With gentle words,
    the answer be,
        all wrath will turn away.
              —*George Richardson*

Biblical Inspiration: Proverbs 15:1

🌸 Aunt Gertie Strikes Again 🌸

Talk about a stressful day! I was with Aunt Gertie again. I tried to control what I said because it would only make matters worse, but . . . my emotions were over the top!

I've heard that when you're angry you need to write down your feelings or write a letter and then tear up the paper and throw it away. It's supposed to be a great stress reliever, so that's exactly what I did.

When you're angry . . .
write a letter . . .
and throw it away.

Dear Aunt Gertie,

Today was a difficult day. I arrived at your house with good intentions, and I left with my head down and my body barely able to move. I brought you a loaf of my lemon bread, and I planned to wash your windows because I know how much you have always enjoyed your house after a spring-cleaning.

Instead of having a great day together, it was ruined by your continued bickering over the littlest things. Your tongue was like a whip that lashed out time and time again. I'm carrying the scars, not physically, but emotionally. The bread was too tangy; the texture was too coarse. The windows were too streaked and smudged. Your comment about "if you can't do it right, then why do it at all" really hurt my feelings. You even commented on how bad I looked today and said if I'd lose some weight I'd look better.

I have plenty of things to do to fill my days, and I certainly don't need the hassle of your nit-picking that you seem to thrive on. I'm trying to understand what's happening to you, but some days are harder than others. I still love you, Aunt Gertie, but you're making it very difficult to do so!

Your niece,
Sarah

Anger absorbs the very energy that we need to use in challenging circumstances. Anger, blame, and guilt can chain us, and Satan loves this. When we acknowledge this JOY-robber, then we can find relief as we pray for God's assistance and ask for His forgiveness.

> Anger absorbs the very energy that we need to use in challenging circumstances.

Dear Caregiver, Music has a way of wrapping around your heart and binding up the ache. Find what works for you, and use it to bring serenity into your life.

Annetta and Karen

Intimacy with God begins with listening to His voice, but the relationship bursts into full bloom when we move to obey.

—Elizabeth George

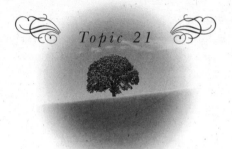

Listening

Dear God,

I certainly don't feel like I'm doing anything worthwhile
   when I go to check on my aunt.
   All she wants me to do is sit down and visit.
   And she really, really loves to talk!

I could be *doing* a lot of helpful things for her instead of
   just sitting.
   I know it's painful when she sweeps. Doing laundry is
      hard on her back.
   But no, she tells me that those things can wait for
      another time.
   I feel so useless!

Honestly, I get restless doing nothing while she repeats
   herself over and over.
   That anxiety leads me to finish her sentences.
   Then I feel guilty because I don't like people doing that
      to me.
   Forgive me, Father.

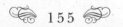

I love her dearly. I want to show her that love.
   She took such good care of me when I was growing up.
   How can I communicate that love when she won't let
   me *do* anything for her?

I'm listening . . .

> ***I love You,***
> ***Your Go-getter Child***

Then Jesus said, "He who has ears to hear, let him hear."
—Mark 4:9

Listening

My Child,

If you only knew the wonderful way that you are already
showing your love and
    doing something that validates her worth and helps
    with her healing.
    You are *listening*! This skill is readily available but, at
    the same time, so elusive.

Don't always think that I will give you "big" things to do.
    My Son, Jesus, wrapped a towel around his waist and
    washed his disciples' feet.
    His humble touch connected their hearts.
    Your loving touch of listening does that, too.
    That's the best gift, dearest one, that you can give
    anyone who is suffering.

Job's friends sat and listened to
    him. In fact, they sat with
    him for seven days

    and seven nights and did
    not say *one* word to
    him.

Listeners are like
human journals. … It's
a way to release stress.

    It was when they stopped
    listening that problems
    occurred.

Listeners are like human journals.
    A journal accepts every word that you write, uncondi-
    tionally, and
    gives you the opportunity to vent without being
    criticized.
    It's a way to release stress.

I'm *your* caregiver. As you enJOY My presence, always
    remember that

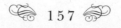

I'm *never* too busy to listen. Absolutely nothing is too unimportant to tell Me.

Be honest with Me! Don't be phony. Go ahead and unload those caregiver emotions.

Vent your frustrations and fears. I forgive you. I can take whatever you dish out!

I will *still* love you forever! That's why I will *always* listen for your voice.

I love you,
God

My dear brothers, take note of this: Everyone should be quick
to listen, slow to speak and slow to become angry.
—James 1:19

Today, walk in the JOY of God's Word!

Read about Jesus washing his disciples' feet in John 13:3–5.

Then they sat on the ground with him
for seven days and seven nights. No one said a word to him,
because they saw how great his suffering was.
—Job 2:13

Let the words of my mouth and the meditation of my heart be
acceptable in your sight, O LORD, my rock and my redeemer.
—Psalm 19:14 ESV

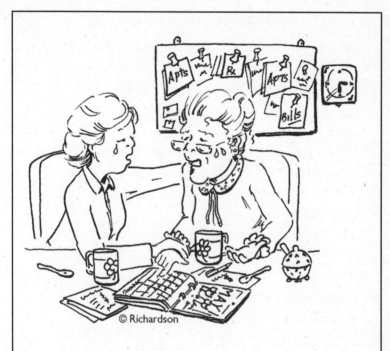

To Live

To live a life of love,
   as Jesus did for me,
no greater way is known,
   or offering so sweet.
     —*George Richardson*

Biblical Inspiration: Ephesians 5:1–2

🍃 Listening, a Gift to Give 🍃

Psychologists say that one of the greatest things we can do for another is to listen. That's giving a heart full of understanding, even if it's filled with laughter and tears.

L **Lock your lip**. Because of anxiety, you may talk more than usual. God gave us *one* mouth and *two* ears for a reason. Use Active Listening Skills:

🍃 Make eye contact.
🍃 Nod head for encouragement.
🍃 Reach out and touch their hand, if appropriate.

I **Insert Prayer**. Pray *for* them and *with* them. Before you pray, ask:

🍃 "How would you like for me to pray for you?"

S **Secret Detective**. At times you need to be a fearless advocate for your loved one and share the things you learn from them with the medical professional. For example:

🍃 Is this a new pain or one that you have experienced before?
🍃 On a scale of one to ten, what is the severity?
🍃 Does the pain occur after eating?
🍃 What usually makes the pain subside?

T **Touch.** We are all born with a great need for touch. Older people are touch-deprived. They are often alone, and their skin dries with aging. The need to be touched increases during periods of stress, illness, loneliness, and depression. Occasionally, reach out and lightly touch their forearm, hand, or shoulder. Through touch they receive . . .

- reassurance and
- a sense of security.

E **Execute open-ended questions to gain information**. Good questions and knowing how to ask them can gather a lot of information. At times they can open gushers of tears, but then healing begins. Open-ended questions require more than a "yes" or "no." Here are some examples of how and how not to ask questions:

- Open: How can I help you?   Closed: Do you need help?

- Open: Where do you hurt?   Closed: Do you hurt?

- Open: What makes the pain go away?   Closed: Does anything help?

N **Notice their body language.**

Watch their emotions and nonverbal communications.

- How do they hold their body?
- Do they make eye contact?
- Do they exhibit tension?
- Are they fidgeting?

Dear Caregiver, What a blessing to have family and friends who listen to us! Make a point to personally thank your family and friends for this blessing. When will you do this?

Annetta and Karen

Loneliness

Dear God,

Even though my daily routine keeps me busy, I hadn't
  anticipated how lonely I would feel.
  I can certainly relate to the lonely-looking sparrow
    standing in my driveway.

As a couple, we always loved having friends come to our
  home for a meal or to play cards.
  As his health declined, I was afraid to invite them.
  I never knew what he would say or do. I was
    embarrassed.
  Our friends felt uncomfortable. He had no clue.

I hadn't anticipated that even my girl friends would eventually stop calling.
  We aren't contagious! Keeping up with what was
    happening in their lives
  helped give me something to think about during this
    season of isolation.

I also hadn't expected that the monthly lunch and gab-fest
with the bridge club
eventually would not happen. Or, maybe they *thought*
I couldn't get away.
I know many medical appointments fell on that day.
Somehow I lost out, I guess.
They had no idea how much the laughing about the
silly things we used to do
helped me to relax and de-stress from the daily routine.

No one understands how lonely a caregiver can feel, even
in this busy world!
How do I survive and thrive?

I'm listening . . .

> *I love You,*
> **Your Child Who Needs a Friend**

Turn to me and be gracious to me,
for I am lonely and afflicted.
—Psalm 25:16

My Child,

Oh, my child, there is nowhere you can go that I won't be
with you.
   If I keep My eye on the smallest birds of the air,
   don't you think that I will keep My eye on you and
      care for you?

I made man for intimacy and companionship because I
never wanted man to be alone.
   Even *before* sin entered the world, I declared, "It is not
      good for man to be alone."

Yes, being a caregiver can be lonely at times.
   Your loved one now isn't the same person you have
      been living with for so many years. You're feeling
      that deep longing for things to still be the same.
   In addition, your friends are trying to come to grips
      with what's happening to you both.

Come to Me. The JOY of my presence will give you
comfort.
   Jesus told His disciples that they would all leave him
      and "scatter,
   each to his own home," but My Son knew I was with
      Him and
   would never leave Him. This gave *Him* comfort.

Paul, in his second letter to Timothy, mentioned that
everyone deserted him
   at his first defense hearing. His way of coping in prison
      was writing
   letters to his friends and the new followers of Christ.

Just as Paul reached out to others, I encourage you to reach
out, too.
  Because of our intimate relationship, your heart will be
    strengthened
  as you endure the lonely seasons.
  I am always with you and will fellowship with you
    throughout the day.

I love you,
God

. . . God has said, "Never will I leave you;
never will I forsake you."
—Hebrews 13:5

Today, walk in the JOY of God's Word!

And the LORD God said, "It is not good that the man should
be alone; I will make him a helper fit for him."
—Genesis 2:18 ESV

Then everyone deserted him and fled.
—Mark 14:50

When you [Timothy] come, bring the cloak that I left with
Carpus at Troas, and my scrolls, especially the parchments.
—2 Timothy 4:13

At my first defense, no one came to my support,
but everyone deserted me. May it not be held against them.
—2 Timothy 4:16

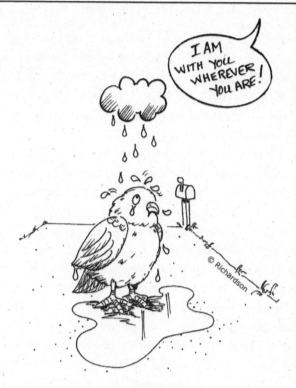

Fly With Me

Things are kind of lonely.
>My life is rather wet.
Caregiving isn't easy,
>but I won't give up yet.
His eye is always on me,
>without a beak in sight.
We will fly together.
>He cares for me, that's right!
>>—*George Richardson*

Biblical Inspiration: Proverbs 18:24

❧ I Tried It. Have You? ❧

Through the nursing home window I watched birds come to eat at the bird feeder outside my husband's room. But my attention was caught by the little bird sitting all alone on a tree branch about twenty feet away. He would only come to the bird feeder when all the others were gone, and then he would fly back to the same branch to sit.

"Yes," I thought. "That's exactly how I feel. Lonely. My husband sleeps most of the day, and when he's awake, he only stares at the ceiling. How I long for just a look from him to say, 'I know you're here.'"

Pastor John arrived and greeted us. After his prayer he commented, "Isn't it enjoyable to watch the birds come to the feeder?" I explained how I was especially watching the one little bird that seemed to be so alone. He brought a chair over to the window where I was sitting, took my hand, and then asked, "How are *you* doing, Lois?"

I'm not sure if it was the gesture of taking my hand or his heart-felt words, but I started to cry. With a trembling lip I said, "I . . . am . . . so . . . lonely." As I wept, I told him how I felt like the little bird who sat on the branch all alone. "My friends haven't been to see me in such a long time—not even a phone call. I don't know whether they don't know what to say or don't want to bother me. Maybe they're not sure if they should talk about my husband's accident, but I'm still me, and I really need my friends! If only they knew how lonely I am!"

Pastor John listened intently. "Lois, you know that you're never alone. God is with you *every* hour of *every* day. When we feel most alone, He will give us what our hearts most long for, comfort and JOY. However, your situation is different from the little bird sitting on that branch out there. Perhaps he's making a choice to come to the feeder alone and not share fellowship with the other birds. Don't make that *your* choice,

Lois. Perhaps you could think of ways to step forward with a kindness for someone else while you're here. Just think about it." We prayed together, and then he left.

Later that afternoon I decided to get a cup of coffee. I noticed a woman at the coffee machine whom I had seen several times before. Remembering Pastor John's words, I took a deep breath, walked over, and introduced myself. It only took a few minutes to find that we had much in common. We even lived in the same neighborhood!

Before going back to our husbands' rooms, my new friend said with a tear in her eye, "How nice it is to be able to talk to someone. I had been feeling so . . . lonely."

Dear Caregiver, Your loneliness can be channeled to be a blessing to others. Try these ideas:

- Ask someone who seems to be alone, "What's the best thing that has happened today?"

- Remember the hard-working staff with a balloon at the nurses' station.

- Tuck a note in a plate of brownies that says, "I appreciate all you are doing for my loved one. Thank you!"

Be alert to the way God surprises you and fills your days with unexpected gifts to remedy your loneliness. Drop us a note at joy4caringhearts@gmail.com, so we can share your "God surprises" with others in the *Nuggets of Hope,* a newsletter for caregivers.

Annetta and Karen

Feeling guilty doesn't *make* me guilty. Feeling guilty means an emotion has attached itself to me. That realization made me a better caregiver, and I was able to focus on the more positive things in life.

—Cecil Murphey

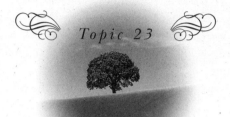

Long-Distance Caregiving

Dear God,

People who think that long-distance caregiving gives you
  some kind of immunity
    from feeling overwhelmed by what is happening to
      your parents are wrong!

I may not be physically exhausted from the daily, hands-on
  caregiving,
    but I still feel worried, anxious, and oh, so *guilty*!

I feel *guilty*
      . . . when I'm with my mom and dad
          because I'm not with my own family, taking care
            of them.
      . . . when I'm at home
          because I'm not with my aging parents.
      . . . because I must depend on their neighbors to be
        my eyes and ears
          and to provide a realistic view of what is going on.

I am so thankful that I am able to drive that long distance once a week,
   but I feel *guilty* about trying to complete their "to do" list,
   and I just never take time to listen to them.

As I wave "goodbye" to them, my tears start flowing.
   I'm scared to leave them alone.
   I'm sad that life is changing so rapidly.
   And I'm praising You, Lord, for keeping them in Your care.

Thank you, Lord, for loving me.
   Please help me through the challenges of the sandwich generation!

I'm listening . . .

> *I love You,*
> *Your Guilt-ridden Child*

The LORD will guide you always; he will satisfy your needs in a sun-scorched land and will strengthen your frame.
—Isaiah 58:11

My Child,

Most long-distance caregivers feel guilty about almost everything—
not living closer, not doing enough, taking time off from work.
I understand your concerns and feel your burden.

Even the early Christians were
concerned for My servant
Paul while he
was in prison and offered
their long-distance
support.

Caregiving, especially
from a distance, is
likely to bring out a full
range of emotions, both
positive and negative.

Jesus was a mobile caregiver.
He understands what
you're going through
and offers comfort in
your lonely experience.

Caregiving, especially from a distance, is likely to bring out
a full range of emotions,
both positive and negative. For loved ones who need
special care at this stage in life,
it is important to be sensitive, involved, and committed.

Feel the blessings that come with:

- working together to know where legal papers are in case of an emergency.
- the modern technology that allows you the freedom to keep in touch.
- establishing a closer relationship with family members.

Affirm yourself for the types of care you provide for your
loved ones from a distance.
> Rely on My love and guidance in caring for your loved
> ones and for yourself.
> Do not lose heart. I love you and will take care of you.

You will find that I will give you the hope that will put
JOY back in your heart.
> The more you are rooted in Jesus Christ, the more you
> will feel like rejoicing!

I love you,
God

Trust in the LORD with all your heart and do not lean on
your own understanding; in all your ways acknowledge him,
and he will make your paths straight.
—Proverbs 3:5–6

Today, walk in the JOY of God's Word!

Let your face shine on your servant;
save me in your unfailing love.
—Psalm 31:16

Cast all your anxiety on him because he cares for you.
—1 Peter 5:7

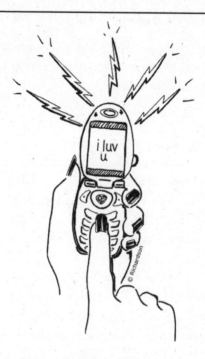

Sending Love

I talk to God,
    He answers me,
        and so it is with you.
I send you thoughts,
    and you reply,
        our meetings are so few.
But if I find,
    it is His will,
        my time and schedules bend,
I hope to touch
    your hand with love,
        instead of pressing "send."
                    —*George Richardson*

Biblical Inspiration: Proverbs 19:21

❧ Challenges and JOYS ❧

We hope that these excerpts from interviews with two long-distance caregivers will encourage you that seasons change, and there are showers of blessings.[15]

Challenges:
Cate—"After my sister, who lives 900 miles away, was able to share in taking care of Dad, I was a little concerned as to whether she had the patience that was needed. It's been said that you think no one else can do it like you can, but I was relieved to find that Dad was in good hands. 'Sharing' Dad gave my sister and me common ground, and we became even closer."

Ron—"My situation was challenging because my out-of-state aunt only had my sister and me as family. Her Power of Attorney was with her lawyer's secretary because she wanted to stay in her home near her church and friends. She had been taken to another facility, and we hadn't been told. The old facility didn't want to give out any information because of the HIPAA act. I learned that the person who has the Power of Attorney is the only one the facilities contact. Another learning experience!"

JOYS:
Cate—"Even though we all knew that Dad didn't want to 'just be kept alive,' the most difficult thing I had to do was to say 'OK' to hospice care. I hadn't expected how difficult that would be; however, I think it was because at that moment I knew we wouldn't be together much longer. My church family and time with God became even more vital. God seemed closer to me than ever before during that time. That will always be a JOY in my life."

Ron—"My aunt loved to hear my stories about being a teacher because she herself used to be one. She would laugh, give a 'knowing' nod, and be so attentive to everything that I would tell her. Those were moments of JOY that we shared, and I knew she would think about those stories long after I had left."

Dear Caregiver, Being observant when you make your visit will give you clues as to the progression of physical and mental limitations that your loved one might be feeling. Observe:

- a change in physical appearance.

- whether or not your loved one is more confused than during your last visit.

- whether or not the cupboards and refrigerator are stocked with nutritious foods.

- whether or not unpaid bills are lying around.

- if the house is clean and tidy.

In addition, having a phone book from your parents' neighborhood can be helpful for finding state and local services available in your parents' hometown.

Annetta and Karen

God will give you the grace, all the help, and all the emotional strength you need—not only to make it through your struggles, [dear caregiver], but even to smile at them.

—Dale Crawshaw

Memories

Dear God,

Oh, Father, you and I both know that Mom's condition is
  getting worse.
  I am so sad, Lord.

My stomach flips over when my cell phone rings.
  I'm sad because I know she will be leaving me soon,
  but I have JOY in knowing that she will be with You
    in paradise.

Tears run down my cheeks when I think of the splendor
  that she will
    see and enjoy in her new, heavenly body.
    No more pain!

Christmas was difficult. The robe I got her ended up in the
  suitcase
    of the patient who shared the room with her.
    Mom said, "Well, she needed it worse than I did,
      honey. It's okay.
    My old one has still got a lot of life left in it."

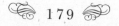

When the time comes, take good care of my mother, Lord.
    Thanks for the many years we've shared together. . .
    even those times when she disciplined me.
    I only tossed the paddle down the clothes chute *once*!

How will I live without her?

I'm listening . . .

> *I love You,*
> *Your Grieving Child*

Jesus said to her [Martha], "I am the resurrection and the
life. Whoever believes in me, though he die,
yet shall he live, and everyone who lives and believes in me
shall never die. Do you believe this?"
—John 11:25–26 ESV

Memories

My Child,

In your mournful season, I am your quiet consolation.
  I am walking with you in the valley, and I am your
    shoulder to cry on.

I, too, have grieved over the loss of a loved one close to me,
    but know, my child, that the splendor of my home is
      like none other.
  The beauty and brilliance is unmatched.
  Its radiance is like a most rare jewel, like jasper, clear as
    crystal.

The old robe of your mother's is one that she loved because
  you gave it to her.
    She has memories of wearing it while she cared for her
      grandchildren.
    I was there with her in the quiet of her hospital room
      as her tears stained
    her beloved robe after she received the news of her
      terminal illness.
    She clung to the robe as she thought back over the
      years of the memories with you. Precious memories!

Remember when the sisters, Mary and Martha, faced real
  life-and-death trouble.
    Their beloved brother, Lazarus, was sick.
    They knew of Jesus' deep love for their brother and of
      his powerful miracles of healing. They sent for Jesus,
      but He did not come right away; and Lazarus died.

When Jesus did come, Martha ran out to meet Him and
  said,
      "Lord, if you had been here, my brother would not
        have died.
      But even now I know that whatever you ask from God,
        God will give you."

Jesus said to her, "Your brother will rise again. I am the resurrection and the life. Whoever believes in Me, though he die, yet shall he live."

Jesus wept with sorrow along with the others over the death of Lazarus.
    His example shows that heartfelt mourning in the face of death does not indicate a
    lack of faith but honest sorrow at the reality of suffering and death.

Remember, nothing can ever take the JOY of the resurrection away.
    It gives hope beyond death.

I love you,
God

For the grace of God that brings salvation
has appeared to all men.
—Titus 2:11

Today, walk in the JOY of the Lord!

Read about the death of Lazarus in John 11:1–44.

Surely God is my help; the Lord is the one who sustains me.
—Psalm 54:4

My flesh and my heart may fail,
but God is the strength of my heart and my portion forever.
—Psalm 73:26

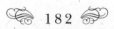

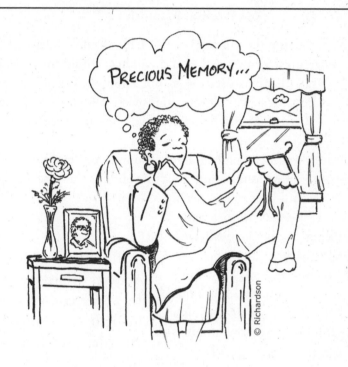

Eternal Moments

This simple robe of memories
        transforms me to the past,
precious days creating
        the moments that will last.

This robe held arms
        that held me close.
She'd smile behind its lace.

And one day we'll meet again,
        as always . . . in God's grace.
                        —*George Richardson*

Biblical Inspiration: John 14:1–4

❧ **Precious Memories** ❧

Walking into the nursing home, I felt chilled and depressed. I wondered yet again how I would find her. Would she be alert or lethargic, happy to see me or not know me? As if waiting for me, her aide's face told me things were not good. She said, "I tucked her into her favorite chair. She's been asleep ever since."

While waiting silently for many hours, my emotions ran rampant. "How long, Lord, must she endure this disease . . . but how can I bear to lose her?"

As I listened to her raspy breathing, I calmed down and thought back to many precious memories—annual vacations to the Great Smoky Mountains . . . helping me with my wedding preparations while she endured bronchitis . . . playing card games with the grandchildren, and oh, how she loved each one of them so much!

Those precious memories helped me to gather my emotions and strength for the final days that lay ahead.

I smiled as those precious memories helped me to gather my emotions and strength for the final days that lay ahead.

Mary, the mother of Jesus, had so many precious memories—the angel's appearance, saying she would bear God's Son . . . the humble birth and visit of the Magi . . . the miracle at Cana when her Son changed water into wine . . . The list could go on and on, but those precious memories sustained Mary through the pain of her Son's death. Imagine her memory of the JOY of His resurrection and ascension. What an extraordinary experience she had!

The JOY from being God's children is more than happiness because it moves us to a different dimension . . . to the JOY of salvation.

Dear Caregiver, Memories are not the key to the past but to the future. Think of five precious memories and talk about these with your friends.

Annetta and Karen

I couldn't make her better or take away the diagnosis. I felt powerless and empty. I did the only thing I could—and I did it for me as well—I prayed.

—Cecil Murphey

Prayer

Dear God,

Every afternoon the kids ask if they can go next door to see
their grandparents.
   I love this time alone, and what a great inter-
      generational time!

Recently I noticed changes
   in my mother-in-law. She
   is struggling with a lack of
   balance,
      and I am beginning a
      caregiving season.

It's not the quick "pray,
eat, and run," but
prayers from their hearts.

But I've also noticed changes
   in the kids' prayers. It's not
   the quick "pray, eat, and run,"
      but prayers from their hearts. At bedtime they now
         include Grandma's special prayer:
      "Now I lay me down to sleep, I pray the Lord my soul
         to keep,

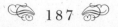

should I die before I wake, I pray the Lord my soul to
take.
*But if I wake before I die, I ask the Lord to show me
why."*

Every time I hear the kids pray that last line, I smile and
overflow with gratitude.
Gracious Father, no matter what our age, you have a
unique purpose for each of us.
Your Holy Spirit is working through my in-laws to
teach us *all*
the JOY and importance of praying.

I was a caregiver for my aunt, so I know the realities of this
season.
Help me to be more diligent in my prayers.

I'm listening . . .

I love You,
A Grateful Caregiver

*Do not be anxious about anything, but in everything, by
prayer and petition, with thanksgiving,
present your requests to God.*
—Philippians 4:6

Prayer

My Child,

I take great delight as I weave surprise blessings throughout
  your day!

Being able to pass their passion for praying down to the
  next generation is very gratifying
    to grandparents, just at it was for Lois and Eunice,
      Timothy's grandmother and mother.
    My plans are always good.
    And I have a *purpose* for each person, *regardless* of their
      age!

My Spirit is at work in your in-laws as their personal
  relationships with My Son, Jesus,
    overflow into the life of your family.
    Because of their rich
      prayer life, you are
      being blessed.

Your desire to have a routine
  prayer time is good,
  but it can't always be
  implemented
    in a caregiver's day,
      when nothing seems
      predictable.
  What is always possible is a *praying life*.[16]

And I (God) have a
purpose for each person,
regardless of their age!

A *praying life* is not limited to a segment of your life or to a
  scheduled event.
    It is an *ongoing* and continual *interaction* with Me.
    There's an *uninterrupted* flow of love between us as
    My Spirit energizes and enlightens your every thought.

Precious caregiver, I love you very much. I'll be waiting for
  you to come into My Presence,

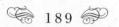

whether it's an established routine or the continual
conversation from your *praying life*.
And, when you think I'm not answering your prayers,
just wait!
Watch to see how I can use disappointments as a
stepping stone for the next victory.
Come into *My* presence, for in My presence, there will
always be fullness of JOY!

I love you,
God

*For the eyes of the Lord are on the righteous
and his ears are attentive to their prayer . . .*
—1 Peter 3:12

Today, walk in the JOY of God's Word!

*The LORD has done great things for us,
and we are filled with joy.*
—Psalm 126:3

*The LORD has heard my cry for mercy;
the LORD accepts my prayer.*
—Psalm 6:9

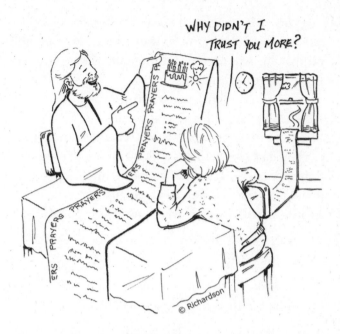

Wise Prayer

"Immortal, invisible,
  God only wise."
Your answers provided,
  seem hid from my eyes.
Your goodness is perfect,
  Your timing is too.
Once I did wonder,
  but now I trust You.

—*George Richardson*

Inspiration: Psalm 84:11–12
and the hymn "Immortal, Invisible, God Only Wise"

🍃 Your Prayer Map 🍃

Have you ever questioned God's timing in answering your prayers? Sarah, Abraham's wife, wanted a child. She indicated to God that she was tired of waiting, and questioned whether or not He was really listening.

Picture in your mind Jesus and you sitting at your kitchen table. And, yes, He will wait until you clean it off. He then unrolls a huge piece of paper that covers the entire table. Jesus looks at you and says, "This is a list of all the prayers you have ever prayed. Look, that's when you were little, and you prayed that it wouldn't rain for your birthday picnic."

You are amazed at seeing every prayer you prayed.

. . . In the ninth grade you wanted your neighbor to ask you for a date.

. . . You wanted a parking spot close to the store. You forgot the handicap sign, and your feet hurt.

. . . You hoped that the lab would call *today* with "good" results.

. . . And this morning, when on your knees, you cried while pleading for endurance to make it through the day.

"Look at how I answered your prayers. Now do you see why I didn't always answer them immediately or the way you wanted? I had something much better planned for you," Jesus says.

Overwhelmed, yet assured of His faithfulness, you look at Jesus and say, "Why didn't I trust You more?"

Satan loves to distort our focus and make us doubt God's promises.

Satan loves to distort our focus and make us doubt God's promises. Look at God's faithfulness to Moses, Naomi, and Job. Trust in His faithfulness to you, too!

Dear Caregiver, Here are two of our favorite tips:

- **Praying Life Coffee Mugs**: Give your loved one a coffee mug just like yours. Use them only during your prayer time. Respect each other's quiet time.

- **Praying Life Gratitude Calendar:** Each day, write down one thing you are thankful for on a dry erase board or calendar. When you have visitors, invite them to write down their word of thanksgiving also.

Annetta and Karen

When you focus on the "what if's" remember that the first step away from your comfort zone in caregiving is stepping into the presence of God.

—Author Unknown

Nursing Home

Dear God,

This decision is breaking my heart.
  I've done everything I could do for the past three years,
  but now it's time—I must relinquish my care to
    someone else.

While the rational part of me knows that this must be
  done for both our sakes,
    another voice inside my head whispers accusations,
    "You are failing your father!"

What if the old, negative stereotypes are true about nursing
  homes?
    I don't want him to be forgotten or uncared for.
    Give him nurses and aides that will treat him with
      dignity
    and respect him as a human being!

What if there is no room for him in the facility I like . . .
  It smelled fresh.
  There is a weekly church service and Bible study, which
    are important to him.
  Give me the wisdom of Solomon to accept that
    wherever there is a room
  for him, it is precisely in Your plan.

It's difficult to discuss this next step with my siblings.
  They haven't had time to help me,
  yet they don't want his money to be spent this way
    either.

Where do I begin, Lord?

I'm listening . . .

> *I love You,*
> *Your Suffering Child*

Blessed is the man who remains steadfast under trial,
for when he has stood the test he will receive
the crown of life, which God has promised to those
who love him.
—James 1:12 ESV

Nursing Home

My Child,

Where do you begin? You begin with the assurance that I
   keep my promises
     and that I have been with your father since he came
      into the world.
     I was with him in the past.
     I will be with him tomorrow.
     And I am with him right now.
     My love for him will *never* change.

I hear the fears of your heart, and I am at work in your
   problems.

Your situation reminds me of Jochebed, Moses' mother.
     She had moments of guilt after hiding her baby and
      then setting him in the bulrushes
   to be cared for by
     Pharaoh's daughter,
   just as you're feeling
     guilty about letting
     your dad be cared for
     at a nursing home.
   She was comforted
     by the JOY of My
     presence in her life,
     and you can be, too.

> I hear the fears of your
> heart, and I am at work
> in your problems.

During the brief time that Jochebed cared for Moses,
     she lovingly nursed her son and diligently trained him
      in the ways of the Lord.
     Your father also has been lovingly cared for by you,
      and I have watched you
     nurture his spiritual life, which I know he appreciates.

Jochebed acted with courage to position Moses inside the
house of Pharaoh.
I used Moses to fight against evil and to save His
people from Egyptian oppression.
You, too, must act with courage in dealing with your
family conflicts.

I love you,
God

Peace I leave with you; my peace I give you.
I do not give to you as the world gives.
Do not let your hearts be troubled and do not be afraid.
—John 14:27

Today, walk in the JOY of God's Word!

Read the story of Jochebed and Moses in Exodus 1 and 2.

This is my comfort in my affliction,
that your promise gives me life.
—Psalm 119:50

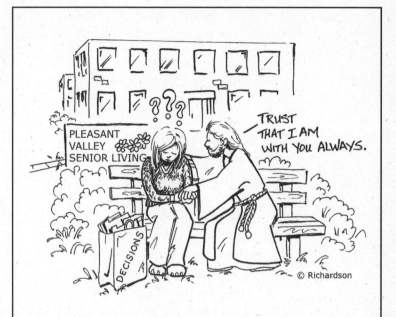

Please Help

When wisdom fails
    and frailty rules
        and fears control the night.
Lord, please help me honor them,
    these children of the Light.

—George Richardson

Biblical Inspiration: Psalm 90:14–17

❦ "Dignity"[17] ❧

I never wanted to end up this way
Helpless to help myself
With the simple day to day
I wish for the time
When good health was mine
I miss who I used to be
And what I miss the most
Is my dignity

When I act hurtful,
It's because I feel ashamed
Broken, in bondage to
This unresponsive frame
I can't tie my shoes
I can't brush my hair
I'm dependent for every need
And no one wants to live
Without dignity

I look in your eyes
And to my surprise
When you look at me
You see more than a disease

It's by your caring
That I am getting through
You have been Jesus
When only He would do
When this is hard

Nursing Home

Know deep in your heart
The gift that you've given to me
That gift is nothing less
Than my dignity

Because of how you love
I have dignity

—Words and Music by Steve Siler

Dear Caregiver, To help in the transition from home to the nursing home, here is a tip: Make an album or scrapbook that is sturdy and can withstand being dropped or spilled on. You could call it *Memories of Joyful Times*. Have each family member write a note of special things they remember about your loved one. Leave the album with them in the nursing home.

Annetta and Karen

The best exercise for the heart is reaching down and uplifting someone with encouraging words.

—Author Unknown

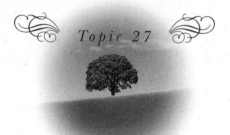
Being Physically Fit

Dear God,

I really like my compassionate doctor. He takes his time
  answering my questions.
    Thanks for this blessing!

I'll never forget the look on his face today when he walked
  in the examination room
    and saw me with yet another family member I was
      caring for.
    He knows that in the past six years I have cared for my
      mother, moved my
    father into my home, and six months later helped my
      daughter after her
    stroke. Her four children needed their grandma.

My doctor assessed his newest patient, my sixty-year-old
  baby sister.
    Then he turned to me, "I'm very concerned about your
      health.
    Are you getting any exercise?"

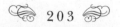

I told him I had a treadmill and a stationary bike. He
  laughed and said,
    "Looking at them does nothing for your health. You
      need to use them!"

Lord, deep within I know I need to take care of myself *now*
    or someone will be taking care of me.
    But exercise? When?

I'm listening . . .

> *I love You,*
> *Your Tension-filled Child*

Do you not know that your body is a temple of the Holy Spirit,
  who is in you, whom you have received from God?
  You are not your own; you were bought at a price.
  Therefore honor God with your body.
  —1 Corinthians 6:19–20

Being Physically Fit

My Child,

I know the *desire* in your heart to get some exercise and
how hard it is to *discipline* yourself to take the time.

Like most caregivers, you have very little control over your
time.
What you can control, though, is choosing to keep fit
and healthy.
The feelings of futility and frustration, common to all
caregivers, will still
plague you, but exercise will keep you resilient!

There are small steps that
can be incorporated *daily*
to improve your physical
fitness.
A little each day will add
up to a lot, and your
body will give back
increased stamina.

Like most caregivers,
you have very little
control over your time.
What you can control,
though, is choosing to
keep fit and healthy.

Some very low-impact movements that help maintain
good mental health and
relieve stress
are deep breathing, stretching, and walking.
These are such a natural part of you that those around
you won't even be aware
that you're exercising! These movements can be done
while sitting at
appointments, watching TV, talking on the phone, or
at bedtime.

JOY-spirations for Caregivers

Dearest child, your body is a good and wonderful gift from
Me.
  It's capable of miraculous feats, if properly taken care
    of.
  It's the temple of the Holy Spirit, who lives within you.
  Value your body by taking good care of My home.

Your physical body is susceptible to disease and injury,
    but faith can sustain you through these crises.
    Having a daily *spiritual workout* in My Word will
    give you strength to rise above the pressures in life.
    Exercising thankfulness is like an adrenaline rush for
      the soul.

No matter what is taking place in your life, there are always
  blessings to count!

Begin today with physical and spiritual workouts to bring
  balance to your life
    and JOY in your caregiving!

I love you,
God

For we are God's workmanship, created in Christ Jesus to do
good works, which God prepared in advance for us to do.
—Ephesians 2:10

Today, walk in the JOY of God's Word!

He will teach us his ways, so that we may walk in his paths . . .
—Isaiah 2:3

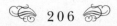

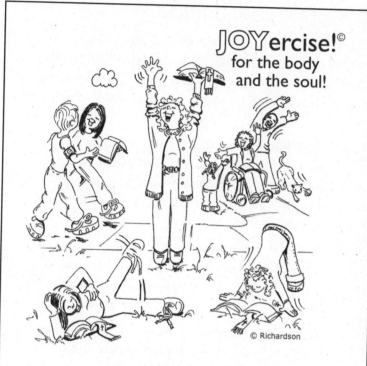

© Richardson

The JOYerciser "Cheer"

JOY-er-ciser! Re-al-izer!
      Stretching is the game!
In His Word! In my walk!
     It is all the same!

JOY-er-ciser! Su-per-sizer!
      Bulking up for God!
Every day! All the way!
      Purposed in my bod!
Hooray! Clapping! Hooray!

—George Richardson

Biblical Inspiration: Philippians 2:12

❧ JOYercise! ❧

JOYercise for the body and soul combines the real JOY you have from your relationship with Jesus Christ with simple physical movements. Incorporate these into the things you already do as a caregiver so you can relax and be rejuvenated!

Breathing: Controlled breathing, taking deep breaths and slowly releasing them, relieves pent-up tension, calms nerves, and helps lower blood pressure. Do this anytime, but make it a habit to do while fixing your morning coffee.

Spiritual Breathing: Stand tall while holding your Bible. Take deep breaths as you read one of God's promises. While exhaling, repeat these words, "Thank You, Lord. Thank You, Lord. Thank You, Lord."

Stretching: Stretching is beneficial for keeping muscles loose and preventing injury as you exercise and provide care. It also releases tension that has accumulated in the muscles. Begin a new habit by stretching before you get out of bed each morning.

Spiritual Stretching: Stretch your arms high above your head, thanking God for the JOY of His everlasting presence. Next, stretch your arms out in front of you and say, "This is the day the Lord has made; let us rejoice and be glad in it" (Ps. 118:24).

Walking: It is good for your entire body. As blood is circulated from your heart to your lungs, the result is more energy. It also contributes to the production of serotonin, which provides an overall good feeling. Choose one of the following to do twice a day for ten minutes: walk around the house or outside, walk up and down the stairs, or exercise your arms using soup cans instead of dumb bells. You'll be rejuvenated!

Spiritual Walking: Walking through God's Word *daily* will always give you a new perspective, whether you read one verse or several. Physically exercising to His Word, by doing what the Bible verse says, is JOY-filling! Try the following:

- Clap your hands all you people .... Psalm 47:1
- You know when I sit and when I rise up... Psalm 139:2
- For you shall laugh .... Luke 6:21
- A little folding of the hands .... Proverbs 24:33
- Why do we sit still? .... Jeremiah 8:14
- Rise up early .... Jeremiah 7:13
- A time to embrace .... Ecclesiastes 3:5

Dear Caregiver, Laughter is jogging for your heart. In case you haven't laughed today, call someone and giggle over anything or nothing at all! Write to us at joy4caringhearts@gmail.com and give us some of your best JOYercise tips! Caregivers would love to read about them in the *Nuggets of Hope* newsletter.

Annetta and Karen

Caregiving is the closest thing we experience to true, self-sacrificing love.

—Terry Hargrave

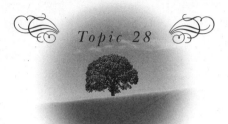

Swallowing Difficulty

Dear God,

What a day this was, Father!

First the nurse came in with medicine to swallow.
He hoarsely told her he couldn't do it.
She replied, "Oh, let's just try."
His eyes held mine with such pleading.
I intervened and explained it all, *again*!

He's tried the swallowing tests, but he hasn't "passed" yet.
There was very little improvement from the last test,
thus he remains NPO (nothing by mouth).

His sister said she was coming to visit right after lunch;
however,
she couldn't get here until almost 5:30.
He was exhausted; I was disgruntled.
There is so much to do (clean and shave his face, dress
him in a clean pajama top,
and time his personal needs to correlate with visitors).

You've seen many of my quiet tears during the last few
  months.
  Life has taught me that I cannot walk this road alone.
  Be with us as our guide, our comforter, and our
    beacon of light.

We cling to the hope that You are in control.
  My husband is in a position of complete helplessness,
  where there is nothing more he can do for himself.
  Is that where you want him, Lord?
  Help me to know your will.

I'm listening . . .

I love You,
Your Nervous Child

In my distress I called to the LORD;
I cried to my God for help. From his temple he heard my voice;
my cry came before him, into his ears.
—Psalm 18:6

Swallowing Difficulty

My Child,

I want you to be strong in Me.
   Yes, I know you don't feel strong now.
   That's why I'm not asking you to be strong in your
      own strength.
   Rather, I'm asking you to
      be strong in Me.

My strength is all-powerful, **When you are weakest,**
   with no limitations. **that is when My strength**
   Your own strength can be **in you is strongest.**
      diminished when you
      are faced with painful
      circumstances.
   When you are weakest,
      that is when My strength in you is strongest.

Look at the strength of these people whom I helped:
   Nehemiah rebuilt the wall of Jerusalem,
   but it's how he humbled himself before Me that is the
      real story.
   Caleb won the right to enter the promised land,
   because his courage and faith rested on his understand-
      ing of Me.

I am your power source!
   ❧ Be encouraging as your husband tries to
      relearn how to swallow.
   ❧ Help him to explain to others—even when it's
      the 77th time.
   ❧ You are a strong caregiver; and I'm by your
      side, cheering you on.

"Do unto others as you would have them do unto you" is a
scripture verse that
you are experiencing first-hand and learning from.
I know that you will pass on JOY, love, and kindness
to those in distress—and
you will be punctual with all of it. You see that it is so
important for your loved one.

I love you,
God

Finally, be strong in the Lord and in His great power.
—Ephesians 6:10

Today, walk in the JOY of God's Word!

Read about Nehemiah in Nehemiah 1–4.
Read about Caleb in Numbers 13–14.

> *[Jesus said], So in everything, do to others*
> *what you would have them do to you, . . .*
> —Matthew 7:12

> *. . . For when I am weak, then I am strong.*
> —2 Corinthians 12:10

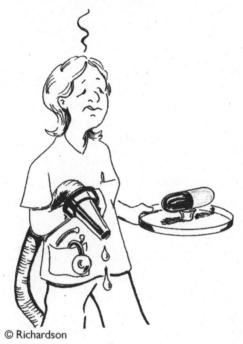

© Richardson

Duty

We all at times resist the good,
  in which His plan provides.
Deliver us, O gentle God,
  through this duty that is mine.

—*George Richardson*

Biblical Inspiration: Psalm 34:17

🐝 Don't Take Swallowing for Granted! 🐝

"After all these years I still have trouble swallowing medicine . . . even something as simple as a vitamin!" My good friend Iris shared this while talking about the years she was a caregiver for her husband, Don. Don had esophageal cancer and was treated with chemo, radiation, and surgery. The surgeon removed his esophagus and pulled his stomach up to create an artificial esophagus. Then Don had to learn to swallow all over again.

Have you ever tried to swallow some medicines, only to have them get caught in your throat? Your reaction is to panic, but common sense says to keep trying to quickly gulp water to get the offending pills down. This is how some people with dysphagia feel every time they try to swallow. For the caregiver, this can be just as scary, because if the loved one aspirates some bits of food or liquid, there is a chance of aspiration pneumonia resulting.

Iris said that she identifies with the widow of Zaraphath (1 Kings 17:8–18) "Don would say to my son and me to take care of each other, trust in and serve the Lord, never stop caring for others, and trust always that the Lord would take care of us. There were situations in the story of the widow that fit our circumstances."

Caregiving can bring great JOY and great frustration on a daily basis. Iris concludes, "I find it absolutely important that once a commitment is made to a patient and/or caregiver that the promise is binding. So much goes into getting the patient ready as well as myself by the appointed time of the visit. The waiting can drag out

> Caregiving can bring great JOY and great frustration on a daily basis.

and tire the patient and set the caregiver on edge. I no longer promise I will be somewhere at a certain time with a shut-in because I don't want to disappoint another."[18]

Don is now with Jesus and suffers no more, and Iris continues to serve others with JOY and Jesus in her heart. Even though there were probably times she felt that she was adrift on the turbulent ocean, God was cradling and holding her and knew the direction of her drift. "But I trust in you, O Lord; I say, 'You are my God.' My times are in your hands" (Psalms 31:14–15).

Dear Caregiver, Friends, visitors, and strangers witnessed the depth and devotion of this family's faith. May you be filled with the JOY of the Lord as you witness your life to those around you.

Karen and Annetta

It's not enough to know God's Word; you've got to take it to heart!

—Christin Ditchfield

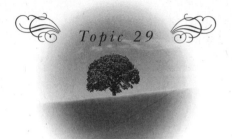

Being in the Word

Dear God,

Help me to figure something out, and do it soon, please.

Why is it that the *urgent* seems to overtake the *important*
    things in life?
        Everything I do seems urgent because people need
            me—now.

Since there are just two of us, I'm on the go constantly.
        My daughter is taking driving lessons. My aging
            parents are facing new limitations.
        It's the busy season at work.
        And even though I get tired more quickly since my
            radiation, I *need* that overtime.
        My dearest friend, who so faithfully helped me, now
            has cancer,
        and I want to be there for her.

Heavenly Father, You know my heart and how desperately
        I want to get back to spending time with You!

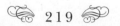

I'm ashamed to admit it, but whenever I need to cut
something out of my day,
It's usually the time I have to read my Bible.
Forgive me! Forgive me!

As a child, I heard my mother say how content she felt and
how much better her days
went after she spent time reading Your Word.
Through the challenges and changes in my life, I've
learned that also.
That's what frustrates me. As a caregiver, how can I get
back into Scripture?

I'm listening . . .

I love You,
Your Frustrated Child

Blessed are those who hunger and thirst for righteousness,
for they will be filled.
—Matthew 5:6

My Child,

You have asked for forgiveness, and that has been done through my Son, Jesus Christ.

As your best Friend, I *cherish* whatever time you spend with Me.

> Any friendship requires spending time together if it is to grow and thrive.
>
> I know how much you enjoy being with your friends, and being with Me is no different.
>
> After all, what kind of friendship would we sustain if we never had time to be together?

Martha of Bethany had that choice to make as she tried to *balance* the urgent and the important.

> Even though she had the privilege of having Jesus at her house,
>
> she focused on the urgent tasks first,
>
> unlike her sister, Mary, who sat at Jesus' feet.
>
> Mary's choice wasn't out of obligation, but devotion!

My Word within you will fill and *restore* your soul.

Jesus didn't tell Martha that work wasn't important but that time *with* Him *must* come first.

> It's from that relationship that she'd be strengthened for *all* other things.
>
> Our relationship is like a waterfall. The top pool first must be filled full in order
>
> to flow effectively into other areas. My Word within you will fill and *restore* your soul
>
> and guide you in all the other areas of your life.

Right now, precious caregiver, is a season when things can't
always be like they used to be.
Life is complicated, so don't lose your desire to read
your Bible.
I encourage you to be creative,
like Zaccheus was when he went out on a limb to be
with Me.
You may not have a lot of time, but you do have some
time.

The JOY of My Word will refresh and revitalize you!

I love you,
God

But seek first his kingdom and his righteousness, and all these
things will be given to you as well.
—Matthew 6:33

Today, walk in the JOY of God's Word!

Read about Zaccheus in Luke 19.

I no longer call you servants, because a servant does not know
his master's business. Instead, I have called you friends,
for everything that I learned from my Father
I have made known to you.
—John 15:15

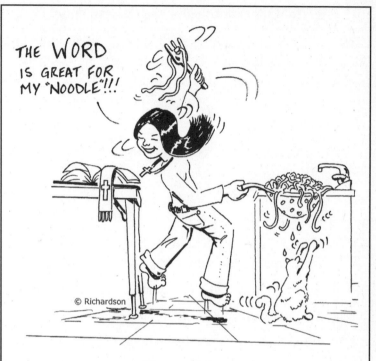

Taste and See

Feeding on the Word of God,
    when I get the chance.
At times I study long,
    but often just a glance.
This culinary outcome,
    from recipe or doodle,
        always claims its starting point
        by what goes in the noodle.

    —*George Richardson*

Biblical Inspiration: Psalm 34:8

✤ JOYful Opportunities for the Caregiver's Soul ✤

The soul's deep thirst, plus the Lord's guidance and a little ingenuity, can help you find a way to welcome God's Word into your busy day. Here are some ideas:

- Display a Bible verse on your computer screen saver.
- Make your computer password your favorite Scripture text.
- When stressed say, "Create in me a clean heart, O Lord, and renew a steadfast spirit within me" (Ps. 51:10).
- Give praise for something whenever you stop for a red light: friends, fresh air, doctors who listen . . .
- Play a Scripture CD when driving in the car.
- Set the radio dial to a Christian station.
- Write one verse of a Proverb on a sticky note and place it on the phone.
- Use a calendar with Bible verses.
- Ask your loved one about his or her favorite childhood Bible story. Then read it together.
- Copy a favorite Bible verse on a file card and staple it to the top of your grocery list.
- Drink from a mug that has a Bible verse printed on the side.
- Place bookmarks with Bible texts by your dinner plate.
- Buy candy mints with Bible verses on the wrappers.

Dear Caregiver, Instead of closing your Bible and keeping it on a shelf, leave it open and lying on the kitchen counter. Read a verse as you walk by. Inhale hope from God's Word then exhale the JOY of His presence. It's also a great witness to whoever comes into your home that God's Word is in use!

Annetta and Karen

What a relief to know that even when I'm restless and can't sleep God lovingly watches over me.

—Author Unknown

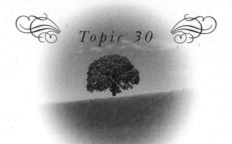

Sleepless

Dear God,

This seems to be a typical morning: when I wake up, my
 back aches and my neck hurts,
  and yet my mind explodes with thoughts—like
   firecrackers on the Fourth of July!
  *Did I pay the last doctor bill? Is there enough money to
   pay it?*
  *Don't forget to put the wheelchair in the car. Oil the
   squeak!*
  I should take time to call my sister . . .

Lord, help me to make it through another day, and help
 me not to be grumpy
  because of my lack of sleep!

Sleeping on the floor by my husband's hospital bed every
 night is my choice.
  I want to do it, even with the backaches and waking
   up tired.
  He could try to get up and then fall.
  Or what if he called out and I couldn't hear him?

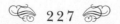

It seems to be a comfort to him that I stay close,
but I can't bump him because that sends pain shooting
down his legs.

I'm heartsick watching my husband fade from me;
yet I praise You for every moment we still have
together.

Lord, every day is a challenge!

I'm listening . . .

I love You,
Your Sleepless Child

Fear not, for I am with you; be not dismayed,
for I am your God; I will strengthen you, I will help you.
I will uphold you with my righteous right hand.
—Isaiah 41:10

My Child,

I'm so glad that you come to Me with your every thought!
　　You can count on My faithfulness to listen
　　and My grace to bring the *real* JOY into your heart.
　　Anytime, anywhere, talk to
　　　Me, and I will listen.

I see how weary you are from lack
　　of sleep and concern.
　　　I saw Jacob with his head on
　　　a rock while he slept, and
　　　I see you sleeping on the
　　　floor.
　　Come to me, and I will give
　　　you rest.

> Anytime, anywhere,
> talk to Me, and
> I will listen.

Do you remember how content Paul was, even while trying
　　to sleep on those sewer-smelling,
　　　damp, cold, rough prison floors?

My face will shine upon you, too, just as it did for Paul in
　　prison.
　　　Trust that my grace will always be sufficient for your
　　　　needs,
　　　even though you may not
　　　　think so at the time.

Let the JOY of my presence give
　　you hope and comfort for your
　　days and nights!
　　　Your attitude of love gives
　　　　your loved one continued
　　　　encouragement
　　　in his pain and suffering.

> Your attitude of
> love gives your
> loved one continued
> encouragement . . .

The world may forget your service as a caregiver, but I will never forget.
When you tend to your loved one's needs, you are doing those things for My Son, Jesus.

I love you,
God

And God is able to make all grace abound to you,
so that having all sufficiency in all things at all times,
you may abound in every good work.
—2 Corinthians 9:8

Today, walk in the JOY of God's Word!

Read about Paul in prison in Acts 16:16–40.

When he [Jacob] reached a certain place, he stopped for the
night because the sun had set. Taking one of the stones there,
he put it under his head and lay down to sleep.
—Genesis 28:12

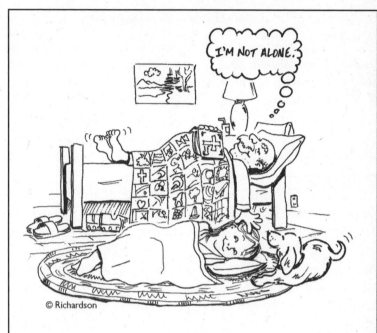

© Richardson

Not Alone

We're not alone,
  His Word assures,
    for God is always there,
      But fear can cause our faith to dim.
May I then work,
  more closely with Him,
    and be forever near.

—*George Richardson*

Biblical Inspiration: John 14:26–27

❧ Good Day . . . Bad Day ☙

I recently overheard three women talking about having a bad day. One said she was grouchy with her neighbors; another was grumpy with her kids. The third added that she had been in a traffic jam, which made her growl at the store clerk. They came to the conclusion that they didn't like being that way, but many things influenced their attitude, especially lack of sleep. Then one said, "I don't really like myself when I feel that way. I don't think anyone else does either."

People say that when they are having a good day in life, they really feel God's love. It's almost tangible. But on a bad day, it's a very different story. Not only do they not love themselves, but also they find it impossible that God would love them. We have so little experience with *unconditional* love—something we do not deserve—that we find it baffling.

Rejoice! Find hope in the fact that God's grace is not dependent upon our performance, nor is it rationed out in proportion to our good and bad days. Whether we have had a good night's sleep on a good mattress or very little because of a hard floor, we can find JOY in God's everlasting presence and strength to endure the day's activities.

God is love. Love is God's mission and His favorite pastime for each one of us! You cannot lose God's love—whether you are rested or exhausted! His love overflows with amazing grace.

Dear Caregiver, Whether it's been a short night or not, praise God in the morning. At the end of the day, thank Him for the best thing that happened to you that day. Your grumpiness will be overcome by the glory of God's grace.

Annetta and Karen

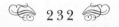

Holidays

Dear God,

It used to be that I looked forward to holidays and
  celebrations!
    But now that Mom is in a nursing home and Dad is in
      a wheelchair . . .
    well, that just puts a whole new perspective on
      everything.

A lot has happened during this past year.
    It seemed like life was just grand, but suddenly our
      lives have shifted,
    in the blink of an eye, to caring for my parents.
    This role reversal *really* scares me!
    It's never going to be the same again, is it?

How will I be able to manage the upcoming holiday
  celebrations?
    I'm already frazzled, and the idea of not having the
      traditional
    home-made Christmas cookies upsets me greatly.

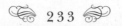

This will be the first Christmas that Mom can't celebrate
   with us at home.
My parents have always been such a big part of our
   celebrations.

This year I'm expected to do it all—do the shopping, clean
   the house,
set the table for eighteen, cook the feast, and take care of
   Mom and Dad, too.
Just the thought of it sends me into a tailspin.

I'm whining, aren't I? But where is the JOY for our
   holidays this year?

I'm listening . . .

> *I love You,*
> *Your Head-spinning Child*

> *. . . Hear my prayer, O LORD;*
> *let my cry for help come to you.*
> —Psalm 102:1

My Child,

You are hurting, and I'm glad you came to me to share the
burdens of your heart.
    I know that the holiday season is such a special time
        for you.
    Yes, you have begun a parent/child role reversal, but
        you will see that
    there can be many blessings associated with this as you
        walk this journey with Me.

Take time for reflection on what
    is most important during your
    holidays.
    Is it how many family dishes
        you can prepare?
    Is it how many gifts you can
        buy?
    Everything doesn't have to
        color-coordinate, does it?

> Take time for
> reflection on what
> is most important
> during your holidays.

Christmas is a time to celebrate
    the birth of My Son, your Savior.
    It's a time to continue your family traditions by taking
        a birthday cake for Jesus
    to your mom and sharing it with others.
    You know how she loves to witness about her faith and
        sing "Joy to the World."

Keep Me *first* in your life, and the *real* JOY of My presence
    will flood your heart
        with comfort and peace.

                    I love you,
                    God

*Praise the Lord. How good it is to sing praises to our God,
how pleasant and fitting to praise him.*
—Psalm 147:1

Today walk in the JOY of God's Word!

Read about the first Christmas in Luke 2:1–20.

*But I will sing of your strength, in the morning I will sing of
your love; for you are my fortress, my refuge in times of trouble.
O my Strength, I sing praise to you;
you, O God, are my fortress, my loving God.*
—Psalm 59:16–17

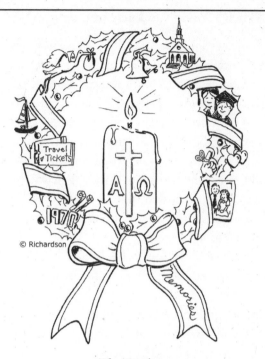

The Light

Thanksgiving, Christmas,
New Year's Eve plans,
how can I manage
with only two hands.
Just let the Light
of the world be the part
you're centered around,
it makes a good start.
And, yes, don't forget
the relationships, too,
while keeping in mind,
My peace is for you.
—*George Richardson*

Biblical Inspiration: Proverbs 17:1

🌿 It's Never Too Early to Celebrate! 🌿

Several years ago, my family celebrated Thanksgiving, Christmas, and my mother's upcoming birthday with my father, who was bedridden in a rented hospital bed set up in the living room. Knowing that he might not make it to the holidays, we included several of our special seasonal traditions. We even decorated his bed to make it look festive.

We played holiday music, and I surprised everyone by putting the old family album on a DVD. A highlight of the day was playing an old video that we had made when we were kids. We laughed until tears streamed down our faces as we watched the silliness displayed onscreen.

Sweet, spicy aromas filled the home, reminiscent of our happy holiday times. Pumpkin pie, homemade cinnamon rolls, and the pungent fragrance of gingerbread with lemon sauce filled the house and seemed to elevate everyone's spirits.

My sister and I went shopping to buy Dad's birthday gifts for Mom. He always gave her chocolate-covered raisins, among other things. It was a tradition and a special memory for them from their dating days.

We sang, and Mom blew out the candles on her gingerbread cake. But we always will remember most the special look that passed between them as she gave him a "thank you" kiss for her gifts.

He died several days later, a month before Thanksgiving, but that last special holiday celebration with him stays in our minds each year.

Dear Caregiver, For many of us, the holiday season wouldn't be complete without certain family traditions that have become the heart and soul of our families. Tidings of JOY and comfort can be yours if you plan ahead. Here are some tips for coping with the holidays:

- ✌ Scheduling celebrations early in the day may be better than having evening festivities.

- ✌ Small gatherings can be more peaceful than large groups.

- ✌ Buffet dinners with many food choices and plate balancing might be too confusing and frustrating for your loved one.

You know best what your loved one can handle comfortably.

Annetta and Karen

The *real* JOY of God's presence fuels our faith to face any obstacle!

—Author Unknown

Unscrupulous Caregiver

Dear God,

Oh, Lord, you have said that you know every detail about me.

>You know my fears and concerns before they're even thought about.

The time has come for in-home care for my step-mother.

>I've heard horror stories about professional caregivers
>
> taking advantage of their clients.
>
> verbally or physically abusing their patients.
>
> deceitfully taking money.

It's agony not knowing which agency to call. This decision is overwhelming.

>I want her treated with dignity and given the "royal" treatment.

Father, you know how difficult it is for me to let go after all this time of caring for her.

>Give me your help so I can make wise decisions for her.

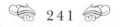

I give you praise each day for being the Way, the Truth,
and the Life
and that brings JOY to my heart.

I'm in a dither, Lord. Whom can I trust?

I'm listening . . .

I love You,
Your Jittery Child

The lions may grow weak and hungry,
but those who seek the LORD lack no good thing.
—Psalm 34:10

Unscrupulous Caregiver

My Child,

The decisions you must make to find reputable people can
be difficult.
> I know how much you love your step-mother. It's
> important to make sure
> that she has the safety, well-being, and care she's
> entitled to.

Yes, there are unscrupulous
caregivers,
> but I want you to know that
> even David once lamented
> to Me that
> his close friend, who came
> to eat at his table, tried to
> hurt him.
> There will always be people
> or situations to guard
> against.

Look closely at the
agencies you may
use, and get second
opinions. Check the
references of all who
enter your home.

Look closely at the agencies you may use, and get second
opinions.
> Check the references of all who enter your home.

Ask your friends to pray for you.
> Pray-ers are your lifeline when you can't seem to take
> the next step.
> The support of your friends in Christ is invaluable in
> helping you
> to walk through this season of life.

In the reign of Herod Agrippa, Peter had been put in
prison for preaching about Jesus.

Herod's plan was to try Peter in public after the time of
the Passover was over.

One of my angels freed Peter from prison. Peter then
went to the home of Mark,

where there was a small group of believers in prayer on
Peter's behalf.

There is power in prayer!

I will always answer prayer. Trust in my faithfulness.

I love you,
God

. . . but God has surely listened and heard my voice in prayer.
Praise be to God, who has not rejected my prayer or withheld
his love from me!
—Psalm 66:19–20

Today, walk in the JOY of God's Word!

Read about Mark and Peter in Acts 12:1–19.

Is any one of you in trouble? He should pray.
Is anyone happy? Let him sing songs of praise.
—James 5:13

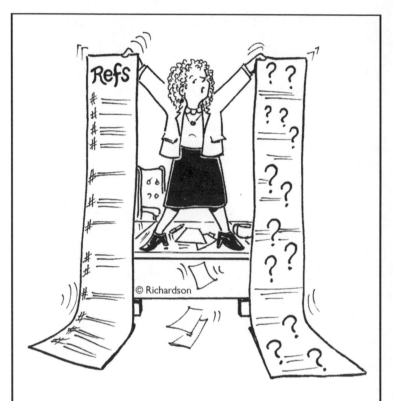

Wise Choice

I want the best
for those I love,
their needs I must provide.
Please grant me wisdom,
and grant me peace,
and referrals verified.
—*George Richardson*

Biblical Inspiration: James 1:5

🐝 Tips for Hiring Professional Caregivers 🐝

Caregiving agencies can be very beneficial to caregivers. Taking care of a loved one in the home can be exhausting for the caregiver, and sometimes the caregiver cannot meet the physical demands.

The list that follows gives some tips you can use when making decisions for in-home care, whether the care is for one shift or round-the-clock:

- Get referrals from hospice for bonded caregiving agencies that they know to be reliable and recommended by their clients.

- Talk with the manager of the agency about how he/she checks the employees' credentials and references.

- For those individuals who will be caring for your loved one in your home, ask the manager about the references for each individual coming into your home.

- Don't be afraid to ask the professional caregiver good questions about your loved one's health. Ask *specific* questions, such as, "What was served for lunch today?" or "How much did my loved one eat?"

- Be aware of your loved one's emotional well-being so you can pick up on unusual panic, worry, or alarm.

- Talk with your loved one about how he/she likes the professional caregivers. Sometimes the personalities of some will connect, while others will not.

- Use open-ended questions when talking with your loved one, such as, "Tell me about your lunch today," or "What did she have you do while she made your bed?" This will help you to assess what is going on during the time you're not there.

Rely on friends to help you make good decisions about in-home care. Often they will have tips from first-hand experience or will know of someone who has been through what you're going through.

Dear Caregiver, Think of the friends in the Bible who shared their hurts and concerns with others. God sent Mary to Elizabeth, Ruth to Naomi, and David to Jonathan. Their relationships show us how close friendships can be. That support is so important. Who are your trusted friends who will pray with and for you?

Annetta and Karen

In my eyes you automatically win the title of hero.

As a caregiver, you are doing the work of the Lord.

When Jesus sees you doing unpleasant tasks for your loved one,

He deems it precious.

You are fulfilling what the Lord said about true, deep love.

—Stacie Ruth Stoelting

Alzheimer's Challenges

Dear God,

Forgetfulness seems to be our *new normal.*

    Just today she forgot how to get dressed.

    I found her sitting on the edge of the bed with a look of "why am I here?"

At the grocery store I said, "I'll be right back; just stay here."

    When I came back, she was gone.

    I was so concerned that she would wander out of the store and into traffic.

    Help me, Lord, to be more responsible in keeping her safe.

Later, I was dozing in my rocking chair, when suddenly I awoke to a burning smell.

    Food was burning on the stove! *Where is she? What happened?*

    I raced through the house, pleading with You to help me find her,

    while asking forgiveness for letting this happen.

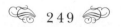

I feel so guilty!
> I feel like a sentinel on 24-hour guard duty. Both times
>> I found her,
> but I can see that I am
>> failing in my responsibili-
>> ties to keep her safe.
> It's really wearing me down.

I feel like a sentinel on
24-hour guard duty.

What can I do?

I'm listening . . .

> *I love You,*
> *Your Guilt-ridden Child*

But I call to God, and the LORD saves me. Evening, and morning and noon I cry out in distress, and he hears my voice.
—Psalm 55:16–17

My Child,

I hear your restless heart, and I know about your feelings of guilt,
  anxiety, and helplessness.

Yes, My child, you are forgiven. Never stop pouring out your overwhelmed heart to me!

Satan will flood your mind with doubt, discouragement, and despair.
  He will do everything he can to make you feel less than you are
  and ill-equipped for the job.

Through your weakness you can rely on My faithfulness!
  Daniel prayed on his knees three times every day.
  He was faithful, even when others plotted against him
  and he knew his life was in jeopardy.

> Satan will flood your mind with doubt, discouragement, and despair.

Rejoice in the opportunity to ask for help.
  That is not showing weakness, but strength!
  Be open to letting Me work through others to help you in your life.

Talk with your family, and share all the things that are happening now.
  It's important that your family members know *exactly* what's happening,
  not only with your loved one but also with you.
  Include them in the decisions that will need to be made.

Rejoice in the unexpected ways I respond to your needs. It
may be
> . . . a friend from church offering to sit with your wife
> while you go shopping.
> . . . a grandchild bringing a meal that all three of you
> can share together.
> . . . a friend stopping by to take you and your wife out
> for ice cream.

The *real* JOY of my presence is *constant*.
> It stays and weathers the shocks of life because I stay
> with you always.

I love you,
God

So do not fear, for I am with you; do not be dismayed,
for I am your God. I will strengthen you and help you:
I will uphold you with my righteous right hand.
—Isaiah 41:10

Today, walk in the JOY of God's Word!

Read Psalm 121, which expresses assurance and hope in
God's protection both day and night.

For I am the LORD, your God, who takes hold of your right
hand and says to you, Do not fear; I will help you.
—Isaiah 41:13

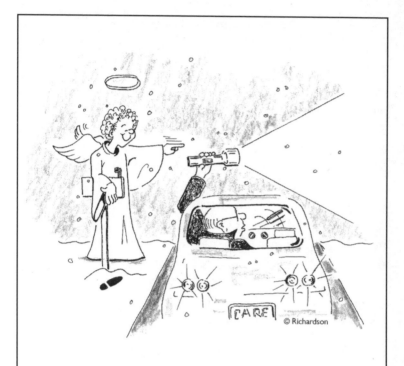

Love the Restless

Help me love the restless,
      who search for what was lost,
steadfast as the Son of Man,
      who seeks the same for us.

—George Richardson

Biblical Inspiration: Luke 19:10

❧ Footprint in the Snow ☙

On a cold, wintry night I was awakened by the slam of the front door. My wife was missing from the bed. I ran to the door to see if I could see her. She was gone. Alzheimer's disease was taking its toll, and she seemed to have a need to walk and walk and walk, especially in the middle of the night. I hurried to put on my heavy winter coat. Finding my car keys seemed to take forever, knowing she was disappearing farther into the night. My wife was seventy-seven, but she could move fast.

I started the car and drove to the end of the driveway, but which way should I turn? Peering into the night, I couldn't see her. I pleaded, "God, please help me find her. Which way did she go? Left or right?" Just then, in a patch of remaining snow, I saw a footprint pointing to the right. I breathed a silent prayer, "Thank You, Lord, for a clue to help me find her. Surround her with your angels to keep her safe."

I turned right, out of the driveway. I drove slowly and carefully, looking on both sides of the road. I found her, still walking, almost a mile from home with no coat to keep her warm. I quietly coaxed her into the car, and we headed home.

As I drove the short distance, my emotions were racing as if they were in a blender on "mix." I was crying silently and shaking from the relief of having found her. I was so afraid I wouldn't and was pleading for guidance so I would know how best to keep her safe.

I keep reminding myself to just take *one* day at a time. My hope is in You, Lord. Thank you for Your special guardian angel watching over her.

Dear Caregiver, Alzheimer's takes its toll on the family, and family members grieve the loss of their loved one. There is JOY in keeping him or her at home, but there may come a time when professional help is needed, both for his or her sake as well as for yours. For now, putting a bell or small alarm on the doorknob could add more weeks to your loved one's home stay. (It worked for Karen.)

Annetta and Karen

There are times in life when all of us are called upon to make heart sacrifices, when we choose to relinquish control and honor. We have to decide to let go. As much as I don't like the process, I am learning that the cup of sorrow can also be a cup of JOY. I believe God's great invitation is to engage us in the process of discovering the power of choosing faith when that decision makes no sense. There is hidden power in our unthinkable circumstances.

—Carol Kent

Decisions

Dear God,

We have some heavy decisions to make, Lord.
> My wife and I need to make decisions about the
> options for her hip replacement. Complicating this
> is her diabetic condition as well as her congestive
> heart failure.
>
> With these multiple medical issues, the decision-
> making on the hip is foggy at best.

There are many risks involved, and the outcome is
unknown.
> The benefits are there, but at what cost?
> This is all creating a confusing maze.

I know we should trust You to help us in all of this.
> I wish you were sitting here right beside me, telling me
> what I should do
> and giving me words to say to my wife.
> She's counting on me to make the right decisions.

I ask your assistance in lifting the fog and
    helping me to be sharp in determining the best way to
    go.

Also, when I am making decisions like this with family
    members,
    I pray that You will give me the wisdom of Solomon,
        the patience of Job,
    the boldness of Peter, and the prayer life of David.

I'm listening . . .

> *I love You,*
> *Your Foggy-headed Child*

> *My heart says of you, "Seek his face!"*
> *Your face, LORD, I will seek.*
> —Psalm 27:8

Decisions

My Child,

You are right to bring Me your concerns about the decisions
you're having to make.

> I love you! I don't love you as a caregiver first;
> I love you because you are My child!
> I desire nothing more than to be with you to bring
> JOY to your hurting heart.

Gideon had decisions to make also.

> I wanted him to defeat the Midianites. Even though I
> promised Gideon that
> I would give him the strength and tools that he
> needed, he still made
> excuses.
> Gideon was seeing only his
> limitations and weaknesses.

Was it easy for Gideon to take
only 300 men with trumpets,
torches, and jars against the
Midianites as I asked him to
do? No, it wasn't! But My
decisions are always for
good.

I (God) understand
the agony you
experience as you
make these types
of decisions.

I understand the agony you experience as you make these
types of decisions.

> I understand because I made the decision for My Son
> to die on the cross
> for the good of mankind. It was agonizing to watch it
> unfold,
> and I will never forget it. But that gift of grace was
> absolutely for the good of all.

Trust me with Your plans. I will continue to go before you to prepare the way. Trust me!

I love you,
God

[Moses said,] "The LORD himself goes before you and will be with you; He will never leave you nor forsake you. Do not be afraid; do not be discouraged."
—Deuteronomy 31:8

Today, walk in the JOY of God's Word!

Read about Gideon in Judges 6 and 7.

How great is the love the Father has lavished on us, that we should be called children of God! And that is what we are!
—1 John 3:1

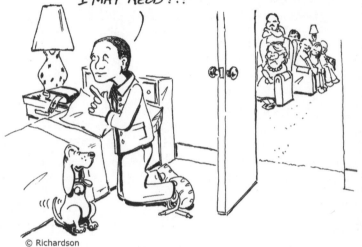

© Richardson

God Knows Best

The Bible says,
  our needs you'll meet,
    in Christ the riches store.
Forget my list,
  Your will be done,
    decisions are a chore.
                    —*George Richardson*

Biblical Inspiration: Philippians 4:19

✿ The Hen and Her Chicks ✿

In pioneer days, wood-burning locomotives frequently sparked fires. Wheat ripens enough to burn ten to fifteen days before it's ripe enough to cut, and sometimes the fires swept wheat fields for ten miles.

A farmer saw billows of smoke in the distance and knew his house, barn, and surrounding buildings were in danger. He set backfires and burned his own wheat fields in a circle so that when the great fire met the place he had burned, it passed around and went on.

With that backfire the farmer saved his buildings but lost his crop. As he walked the burned field grieving, he saw the charred body of a hen. He tipped the hen over with the toe of his boot, and out ran a dozen little chicks. Because the mother's burned body was over them, the chicks lived. She was willing to die so that those under the cover of her wings would live.[19]

The farmer had an agonizing decision to make. Much like the farmer, many times we hurt and don't know where to turn. We reject God's help because we don't think He can give us what we need. But who knows our needs better than our Creator? Those who turn to God for help in decision-making will find that He helps and comforts as no one else can.

Dear Caregiver, "He will cover you with his feathers, and under His wings you will find refuge" (Ps. 91:4). When have you felt yourself under His wings in a crisis? God is good *all* the time! Praise Him!

Annetta and Karen

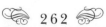

Self-Worth

Dear God,

Worthless! In one word that's how I feel, God. *Worthless!*

It's the same thing day after day.
> Wipe up spilled food from the floor. She wants things
> perfect.
> Try to comb her thinning hair the way she has always
> worn it.
> My rough farmer hands were never meant to do this.
> Serve her coffee at exactly the right temperature, and
> make sure the mug is *hot*, too!

Oh, how I miss having coffee with the men down at the
corner café.
> I miss doing those little carpenter jobs at church.
> That made me feel worthwhile, plus they'd always
> laugh at my jokes.

Now when I do go out, the only thing I'm ever asked about
 is, "How's your wife doing?"
  I respond with a smile, while inside I'm shouting,
   "Does anyone care about me?"
  I feel like an *invisible* person.

There are days I'm grateful and
 feel privileged to be a caregiver.
  Then there are other days
   when I feel so insignificant!
  Lord, I need to be somebody
   that others respect.
  I need to do something
   constructive.

> Does anyone care
> about me? I feel like
> an *invisible* person.

Do other caregivers feel this way?

I'm listening . . .

> *I love You,*
> *Your Worthless Child*

Are not two sparrows sold for a penny? Yet not one of them will
 fall to the ground apart from the will of your Father.
  And even the very hairs of your head are all numbered.
 So don't be afraid; you are worth more than many sparrows.
   —Matthew 10:29–31

Self-Worth

My Child,

Caregiving can be so complicated, because it's a new season of life, with changing
    situations. For you, it's reversing roles with your loved one.

I understand how much you want things to be back to the old routine.
    Changes, like you have experienced, can certainly make you think you have
    no worth, but that couldn't be further from the truth!

Invisible? Never in My eyes!
    I know how many hairs are on your head and how you feel about your receding hairline.
    I know how the arch in your right foot hurts.
    I know that today you are worrying about her loss of strength.
    I know that tomorrow you'll be thankful it is her last chemo treatment.

It's easy, My child, to get so crushed by your circumstances that you can't see yourself
    as I see you—unique, precious, and treasured!

I am a God who will take care of even the tiniest details in your life.
    The Israelites wandered in the desert for 14,600 days, and their feet didn't swell!
    Their clothes never wore out either.
    My constant presence surrounded them as a cloud by day and a pillar of fire at night.

My unfailing love for you didn't begin on the day you were born,
    and it doesn't conclude on the day that you die.

It reaches back into those days *before* you were born, and it reaches ahead into eternity.

Read My Word. Soak up the truth about what gives you worth.
    I sacrificed My only Son, Jesus Christ, for *your* redemption.
    I have summoned you *by name*. You are *mine!*
    Let the real JOY of the Easter resurrection set you free from feeling worthless.

Look in the mirror, and you will see a person of *great worth*!

I love you,
God

See, I have engraved you on the palms of my hands;
your walls are ever before me.
—Isaiah 49:16

Today, walk in the JOY of God's Word!

My frame was not hidden from you when I was made in the secret place. When I was woven together in the depths of the earth, your eyes saw my unformed body. All the days ordained for me were written in your book before one of them came to be. How precious to me are your thoughts, O God! How vast is the sum of them!
—Psalm 139:15–17

Indeed, the hairs of your head are all numbered. Don't be afraid; you are worth more than many sparrows.
—Luke 12:7

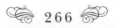

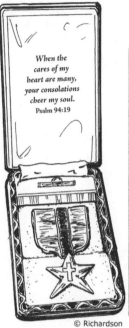

When the
cares of my
heart are many,
your consolations
cheer my soul.
Psalm 94:19

Citation

BY DIRECTION OF
GOD

THE CAREGIVER
MEDAL OF HONOR

IS PRESENTED TO YOU

who distinguishes yourself by outstanding
meritorious service in connection with caregiving
operations under ever-changing situations and in
various seasons of the life of your loved one.

Your loyalty, diligence, and devotion to duty
are in keeping with the highest traditions of the
caregiving service and reflect great credit upon
yourself and the Kingdom of God.

© Richardson

To the Commander

I'm humbled
    that You value me.
I'm honored
    just to serve.
I do not need a medal
    or citation to observe.
I'm grateful
    as your soldier
        to follow as You lead.
The order to love others
    in every word and deed.
        —*George Richardson*

Biblical Inspiration: 2 Timothy 2:4

❧ No, Never! ☙

Crumple a dollar bill. Squeeze it. Put it on the ground. Stomp on it. Roll it in dirt and cover it with mud! Does that bill still have the same value, even after all that?

Yes! Even though its condition changed, the value was *not* lost. It still has its worth!

Moses stuttered. Was he worthless in God's sight? *No!*

Timothy had an ulcer. Was he worthless in God's sight? *No!*

Martha worried. Was she worthless in God's sight? *No!*

Gideon was afraid. Was he worthless in God's sight? *No!*

When you can't get everything done, have *you* lost your value? *No!*

When you ask for help, have you lost your value? *No!*

> When you ask for help, have you lost your value? *No!*

When you are discouraged, depressed, or desperately empty, have you lost your worth? *No!*

When tears come frequently and you feel you've reached the end of your rope and can't face another day of caregiving, have you lost your worth? *No!*

Would Jesus Christ have died on the cross for you if you weren't of *great worth* to Him? *No!*

Can any circumstance be powerful enough that it will separate you from His love? *No!*

When Satan makes you think you are worthless, are you? *No! Never!*

Whenever these negative thoughts of feeling worthless come to you, remember they are from Satan. Whenever he prowls in your mind, just tell him, "No, I'm not going to believe your lies because I'm focusing on the empty grave and risen Christ. That will *never* make me a worthless person!"

Dear Caregiver, Jesus engraved your name on the palm of His hand. "Engraved" means to cut. That hurts! His hands are nail-pierced just for you. Now that's a love beyond all our comprehension, isn't it? Think about this: *If God were describing you to His angels, what would He say?*

(Insert your name in the blank and answer the questions, e.g. <u>Karen</u> has a caring heart. <u>Annetta</u> is an encourager.)

_____ has . . .

_____ is . . .

_____ will . . .

Annetta and Karen

A Sunday School teacher asked if anyone could quote the 23rd Psalm.

A four-year-old raised her hand and then began: "The Lord is my shepherd, that's all I want!"

—Robert Ketchum

Psalm 23

The Lord Is My Shepherd

(To personalize this psalm, write your name on the line)

"The LORD is _____ shepherd, I shall not be in want.
He makes me lie down in green pastures,
he leads me beside quiet waters,
he restores my soul.
He guides me in paths of righteousness
for His name's sake.

Even though I walk through the valley of the
shadow of death,
I will fear no evil, for you are with me;
your rod and your staff, they comfort me.

You prepare a table before me
in the presence of my enemies.
You anoint my head with oil; my cup overflows.

Surely goodness and love will follow me
all the days of my life,
and _____ will dwell in the house of the LORD forever."

🌿 The Lord Is My Caregiver® 🌿

A paraphrase of Psalm 23 by Annetta Dellinger and Karen Boerger

The Lord is my caregiver.
Although I may not feel like I always walk in green pastures,
He is still with me.
He leads me through challenges, tears, frustration, guilt,
and anxiety.
Even though I don't know what will happen tomorrow,
much less today,
because I have no control over it,
I will still walk steadily with Him. He is my refuge and strength.
Oh, how I am comforted when I look to Him!

Satan tempts me as I walk through the valleys of
discouragement and doubt,
but truly I am at peace because I am in my Lord's presence.
His strength is my refuge,
and I rest secure in His arms.

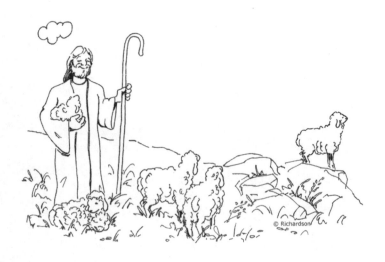

© Richardson

Psalm 23

God fills my days with His awesome love,
and my cup overflows.
His faithfulness through all generations assures me
that His mercies are new each morning, and I can make it
through another day.

My Shepherd, Jesus Christ, died so that all who have been
made new in Him
will no longer live for themselves but for Him alone.
By His grace He leads me through this caregiving journey, and
I will sing praises to Him forevermore.
My Shepherd, My Lord, My Savior, My Caregiver!

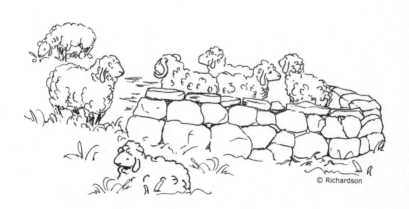

© Richardson

A caregiver is sometimes unknown and often unnoticed,

But you are a hero nonetheless,

For your love, sacrificial, is God at His best.

You walk by faith in the darkness of the great unknown,

And your courage gives life to your beloved.

—Author Unknown

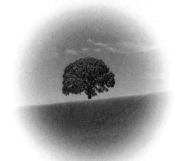

Endnotes

Realities of Caregiving

1. Virelle Kidder, "The Keeping Room," *Donkeys Still Talk: Hearing God's Voice When You're Not Listening* (Colorado Springs, CO: NavPress, 2004), p. 145.

Asking Why Me?

2. Emily Pearl Kingsley, "Welcome to Holland," as published on the United Church of Christ Disabilities Ministries Web site—www.uccdm.org/2000/07/21/acceptance-of-your-child-welcome-to-holland/.

Attitude

3. Judith Viorst, *Alexander and the Terrible, Horrible, No Good, Very Bad Day*, New York: Simon and Schuster, 1987.
4. Author Unknown, "Three Hairs," www.Spiritual-Short-Stories.com.

Trust

5. True Story—Shirley Braddock

Making a Difference

6. Charles Puchta, *Caring for One Another: Biblical Caregiving Principles,* (Aging American Resources, Inc., 2008), p. 94.

Eating Concerns

7. Credit for nutritional information: Carol Lewis, author, speaker, FirstPlace4Health National Director, www.firstplace4health.com and Kathy Loidolt, author and consumer health advocate, www. ShoppersGuidetoHealthyLiving.com.

Equipped for a Purpose

8. Words and Music by Scott Krippayne and Steve Siler, BMG Songs Inc. (Gospel Music Division)/Above the Rim Music/Ariose Music-Administered by EMI Christian Music Publishing, (ASCAP), 1996

Family Conflict

9. Family Conflict Tips contributed by Dr. Catherine Hart Weber, Sierra Madre, CA.

Financial Crisis

10. Financial tips for caregivers contributed by Sherri Goss, Senior Vice President, Rosenberg Financial Group, Inc., Warner Robins, GA, www.myfamilylifebook.com.

Friends

11. "Where's My Help?" by Rev. Bob Willis, Southern Baptist Minister, Bereavement Coordinator for Hospice of Oklahoma County, Grief Recovery Specialist by the Grief Recovery Institute in Los Angeles, Nationally Certified Bereavement Facilitator by the American Academy of Bereavement, and a Compassion Fatigue Specialist through the Traumatology Institute at Florida State University. www.Godhealshearts.com.

Humor

12. Humor insights from Pamela Christian, author/speaker/ radio show host.
13. JOY Boxes—For information on how to create your own unique JOY Box as a gift to a caregiver, contact Annetta Dellinger: www.annettadellinger.com.
14. The Association for Applied and Therapeutic Humor: www.AATH.org.

Long-Distance Caregiving

15. Interviews with Cathy Burns and Ron Gotham.

Prayer

16. Jennifer Kennedy Dean, Bible Study, *Live a Praying Life, Open your Life to God's Power and Provision* (Birmingham, AL: New Hope Publishers, 2003), 11–16.

Nursing Home

17. "Dignity," Words and Music by Steve Siler, Used by permission of Music for the Soul, Inc. and Silerland Music, www.musicforthesoul.org, 2009.

Swallowing Difficulty

18. Interview with Ida Luebke.

Decisions

19. Donald Barnhouse, "The Hen and Her Chicks," *Let Me Illustrate* (Grand Rapids, MI: Fleming H. Revell, 1967), 261.

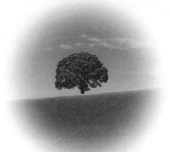

About the Authors

JOYful MINISTRIES

Annetta Dellinger, a JOYologist, is founder of JOYful Ministries. She's a joyburst for Jesus, where inspiration, motivation, and enthusiasm collide. She is known as "the JOY Lady." Her PHD=Perky Happy Disciple.

Annetta is a wife, mother, and grandmother, and has been a spontaneous, spunky, spirit-filled speaker for over twenty years and has authored over thirty books. As an international speaker, she loves working for the Lord, whether it is with small groups, audiences of a thousand, or people on a cruise ship. Annetta's messages are energizing. She motivates her audiences and customizes her messages for different themes. As a leader of women's weekend retreats and a speaker at conventions and workshops, she involves the audience with her power-packed, Biblically-based messages.

The JOY Lady's mission statement is: To encourage and equip women to focus on the real Source of JOY, Jesus Christ, who brings hope in all situations. She serves on the staff of the National SomeOne Cares Christian Caregivers Conferences.

Annetta lives in the Plain City, OH, area with her husband and enjoys spending time with her children and grandchildren.

Contact her for engagements at www.annettadellinger.com.

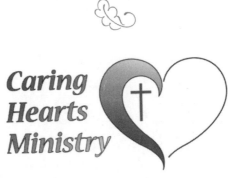

Karen Boerger founded Caring Hearts Ministry to bring hope and encouragement to caregivers. Her mission statement is to energize the caregiver, equip those with caring hearts, and encourage all with the real source of JOY, Jesus Christ.

After twenty-four years in the teaching ministry and six caregiving experiences during that time, Karen felt the need to use her caregiving experiences to help others. She could see God's plan in her life and now wants to share God's love with these silent heroes at retreats, workshops, conventions, and special events.

Karen works with the Caring Hearts committee in her congregation to bring JOY and encouragement to church members in need. Karen also enjoys teaching Sunday school and singing in the choir.

About the Authors

Karen and her husband live in central Ohio on the family farm and enjoy world traveling, movies, football, and nature. They enjoy three children and seven grandchildren that keep them young.

To contact her for speaking engagements or to subscribe to her monthly newsletters for caregivers, *Nuggets of Hope,* visit her Web site at www.karenboerger.com.

[Personalize this message by writing your name on the line.]

Dear Caregiver,

    I am _____ *'s caregiver.*

    My love for _____ *is everlasting.*

Love,

God

For I am convinced that neither death nor life, neither angels nor demons, neither the present nor the future, nor any powers, neither height nor depth, nor anything else in all creation, will be able to separate us from the love of God that is in Christ Jesus our Lord.

—Romans 8:38

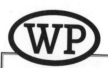